COVID-19:
The Postgenomic Pandemic

COVID-19:
The Postgenomic Pandemic

Hugh Pennington

polity

First published in 2022 by Polity Press

Polity Press
65 Bridge Street
Cambridge CB2 1UR, UK

Polity Press
111 River Street
Hoboken, NJ 07030, USA

ISBN-13: 978-1-5095-5214-6
ISBN-13: 978-1-5095-5215-3 (pb)

A catalogue record for this book is available from the British Library.

Library of Congress Control Number: 2022933625

Typeset in 11 on 14pt Sabon
by Cheshire Typesetting Ltd, Cuddington, Cheshire
Printed and bound in Great Britain by CPI Group (UK) Ltd, Croydon

The publisher has used its best endeavours to ensure that the URLs for external websites referred to in this book are correct and active at the time of going to press. However, the publisher has no responsibility for the websites and can make no guarantee that a site will remain live or that the content is or will remain appropriate.

Every effort has been made to trace all copyright holders, but if any have been overlooked the publisher will be pleased to include any necessary credits in any subsequent reprint or edition.

For further information on Polity, visit our website:
politybooks.com

Contents

Foreword

A virus has been described as an 'astonishingly efficient and beautiful product of nature' because it is so economical in its genetic information, because it attaches efficiently to host cells, because it effectively directs the manufacture of new virus components and genomes once inside, and because it is stable in the environment but still speedily disgorges its internal components into host cells after contact.[1] Inside each SARS-CoV-2 virus, the one that causes COVID-19, is a long molecule made of RNA, its genome. It is surrounded by proteins which enable it to get into the cells lining our noses, throats and lungs, and grow in them. Postgenomics is a convenient term to describe the scientific study in real time of the sequence of the building blocks of that molecule, and the use of that information to detect it, to follow its evolution, to exploit its differences as a fingerprinting tool to track the spread of the virus, and to use it to make vaccines and search for antiviral drugs. The chapters that follow describe the science enabling these endeavours. They are written for the non-scientist.

Foreword

History explains how we got to where we are, and so chapter 1 describes the development of postgenomics since Watson and Crick and DNA in the 1950s. Chapter 2 describes coronaviruses and their discovery, first as common cold viruses and then as very nasty causes of pneumonia; SARS (originally from bats) and MERS (from camels). Chapter 3 is about COVID-19 as an acute disease, its treatments and its chronic complications. The next three chapters describe early events in the pandemic as they happened, starting in chapter 4 with the possible origins of the virus at the end of 2019, favouring a natural rather than a man-made birth; then, in chapter 5, events in February and March 2020, focusing on a comparison of the English Nightingale Hospitals with their Chinese precursors, Fangcang shelter hospitals; and going on, in chapter 6, to the exhortation in March to test, test, test and the big postgenomic spin-off, polymerase chain reaction (PCR). SARS-CoV-2 is not only modern as a new human pathogen, but particularly deadly because worldwide modernity means that we are living longer and getting fatter, the two most important risk factors for lethality, as described in chapter 7. Local outbreaks give vitally important information about factors that help the virus to spread and have driven control policies, and are covered in chapter 8. The benefits that have come from the method that characterizes the postgenomic era, rapid genome sequencing, are considered in chapter 9 and, with others largely dependent on it, the detection and effects of variants, in chapter 10, and vaccines, in chapter 11. Previous pregenomic pandemics are considered in chapter 12; they put COVID-19 into context and lay the historical foundations for the final chapter. There is one Sam Goldwyn quote I use a lot: 'Making predictions is difficult, particularly about the future.' So read its prognostications about what might happen in years to come with scepticism; but do not doubt the importance of luck.

This book is about science. No comment is made about the response of national leaders to the pandemic, or how different nations have coped with it differently, despite it spreading on the air in the same way everywhere, and no comment is made about the impact of that endemic condition, banal nationalism.[2] Social media is avoided like the plague. Most tweets have R numbers many orders of magnitude greater than the fastest-spreading microbes.

No account is free of bias. This one is evidence-based. It relies on scientific papers. It is biased because only a few have been chosen for emphasis out of the vast number that have been published; within the first 10 months of the pandemic, more than 125,000 had been written;[3] and biased because it is an account written by a molecular virologist[4] who has researched virus virulence and virus variants, handled smallpox virus, reverted to bacteriology and investigated *E. coli* O157, a new pathogen that spread worldwide late in the twentieth century, and a scientist who has long held a positive view about the correctness of John Stuart Mill's essay on Nature,[5] one that COVID-19 has abundantly justified: Nature kills and tortures 'with the most supercilious disregard both of mercy and of justice', and the precept that man ought to follow nature is irrational 'because all human action whatever, consists in altering, and all useful action in improving, the spontaneous course of nature'.

I

The Postgenomic Age: Its Antecedents

We are now in the Postgenomic Age,[1] the period that started with the publication of the draft sequence of the human genome in 2000, and has since been characterized by revolutionary technical developments that make it possible for biological research to use whole genome sequencing technologies routinely in real time and draw extensively on the genomic knowledge so generated. COVID-19 is postgenomic because these approaches led to the discovery of its cause, the brand-new virus SARS-CoV-2, the development of the test which dominates the diagnosis of the disease in life, and in death, and the availability of methods to characterize the virus genome in precise detail, enabling the detection of variants in real time and the identification of local, national and international routes of spread, with all these things happening at unprecedented speed. A handful of pneumonia cases were diagnosed in Wuhan in December 2019. Deep lung samples were taken from three of them on 30 December. Exhaustive diagnostic testing showed that the illnesses were not caused by any well-known viruses or bacteria. Application of a central post-genomic method, ultrarapid genome sequencing (often called next generation sequencing), identified the cause as a new virus on 7 January. The genome sequence was published internationally on 10 January, test kits designed using the sequence became available the next day,[2] and vaccine researchers had designed and made their first candidate antigens within a week.

Lots of interesting people have made the discoveries and invented the techniques that have made the post-genomic science that underpins the way we recognize, record, research, respond to and resist COVID-19. Sydney Brenner was one. Son of a Lithuanian cobbler who, in 1910, had emigrated to South Africa and who spoke Russian, Yiddish, English, Afrikaans and Zulu but never learned to read or write, Brenner became a giant of molecular biology (awarded the Nobel Prize in 2002). He shared an office with Francis Crick for 20 years. He played a key role, with the electron micros-copist Bob Horne,[3] in developing negative staining, the electron microscope technique that was used to discover coronaviruses.

Brenner divided biology into epochs. BC was 'before cloning'. AD was 'after DNA'. Before it, everything seemed hopeless. After it, thought could be given to trying to sequence genes to get answers to the question 'How do they fit into the broader picture?'

AD developed into the genomic era. This formally began in 1977, when Frederick Sanger in Cambridge (Nobel Prizes for Chemistry, 1958 and 1980) published the genome sequence of the very small bacterial virus, ϕX174. It has a DNA genome less than a fifth of the size of SARS-CoV-2. Sequencing this single tiny genome in the mid-1970s took many months. Technical progress in this area continued to be very slow. Sequencing the human genome was first proposed in 1984. The Human Genome Project (HGP) started in 1990. It took 23 years and cost $2.7 billion. Its main results were announced 11 days before the fiftieth anniversary of the publication of Watson and Crick's description of the DNA double helix. The initial sponsor of the HGP was the US Department of Energy, based at the Oak Ridge National Laboratory in Tennessee, which had been established in the early 1940s to make enriched uranium as part of the Manhattan Project, the place where Teflon came into its own to protect components from uranium hexafluoride, the viciously corrosive gas used in the half-mile-long plant that separated the uranium-235 isotope (used in the Little Boy Hiroshima bomb on 6 August 1945) from U-238. Proponents put the HGP into the same category as the giant accelerators used in nuclear physics.[4] It was Big Science. The first microbial Big Science exercise was the *E. coli* sequencing project, finished in 1997. It took 6 years and involved 259 scientists. Alvin Weinberg, the director of Oak Ridge, compared Big Science to Notre Dame and the Egyptian pyramids as well as to space rockets and experimental nuclear reactors, and was concerned that while it was necessary, it might eventually turn out to be a pathological contagion because its spread could damage Little Science.[5] For biology, he needn't have worried. Quick and cheap methods were developed in the 1960s for comparing bits of genomes (but not whole ones, yet) that did not use complicated equipment or need large teams of technicians. The methods used electrophoresis, in which nucleic acid molecules were separated in porous gels by passing an electric current across a slab of the gel.

Electrophoresis was invented by Arne Tiselius (Nobel Prize for Chemistry, 1948) in Uppsala. His first apparatus was unveiled in 1937. It was massive – 20 feet long and 5 feet high – very expensive and needed a dedicated operator. It was also very slow, had very poor resolving power and could only run one sample at a time. Its successors are more than ten times faster, use bench-top equipment that can run many samples simultaneously with high resolution, cost a hundred times less, and can deliver top-quality results by anyone after a few hours of training. This technical improvement was paralleled by another one that also began in Uppsala. Tiselius worked in Theodor Svedberg's laboratory. In 1925 Svedberg (Nobel Prize for Chemistry, 1926) unveiled his ultracentrifuge, which generated massive g forces big enough to move big molecules in a controlled way. It occupied two rooms, was driven by an oil turbine, needed a hydrogen supply and vacuum pumps, and, in the words of a US biochemist, Professor Dean Fraser, 'had to be run behind 3-foot-thick walls of reinforced concrete. The scientists who operated them were considered slightly insane. Centrifuges required constant attention . . . explosions were to be expected at fairly regular intervals. The Spinco preparative centrifuge, for contrast, is about the size of a washing machine, and anyone can learn to run it in 10 minutes.' I cut my virological teeth on a Spinco in the 1960s.

Genomics would not have been possible without electrophoresis. However, ordinary DNA molecules, even bacterial ones, are too big to be analysed by it. The discovery of restriction enzymes (Werner Arber,

Dan Nathans and Hamilton Smith, Nobel Prizes for Physiology or Medicine, 1978) was a key development. Bacteria make them for defence against virus infections. They recognize the virus DNA as it enters the bacterial cell as foreign, and cut it, making it non-infectious. The cuts are not random but are made at particular DNA sequences along the molecule, so the cutting generates DNA fragments whose size depends on the DNA sequence. They are small enough to be separated in an electrophoresis gel, giving a pattern of bands like a bar code. Fragments with a particular sequence can be detected by hybridizing them with DNA complementary to them labelled with radioactivity. Called Southern blotting, after Ed Southern, its inventor, the electrophoresed DNA fragments are blotted onto a nylon membrane and then treated with the radioactive complementary DNA. Application of an X-ray film to the membrane reveals the bands of interest. The power of this method was dramatically and publicly demonstrated for the first time when it was used by Alec Jeffreys in 1986 during the investigation of two rapes and murders in the English Midlands.

In 2007–8 there was a revolution. Next generation sequencing (NGS), a catch-all term used to define a cluster of technologies, came in. The Postgenomic Age took off. Whole genome sequencing (WGS) of viruses changed overnight from projects that took years, to routine activities that took less than a day per virus, because the speed and cost of sequencing DNA and RNA molecules and genomes had dropped dramatically, massively outpacing Moore's Law (that the number of components on a microprocessor chip doubles every two years, an annual compound growth rate of 35 per cent).[6] The most telling example of this revolution is its impact on the sequencing of the human genome; today, a human genome can be sequenced in 24 hours at a cost of less than $1,000.

An excellent example of a next generation sequencing technique is nanopore sequencing. It was one of the methods used to discover SARS-Cov-2 in early January 2020 and has been used to sequence many thousands of its genomes since, probably about a quarter of those analysed worldwide. By the application of a small voltage, nucleic acids are encouraged to pass through tiny holes in a membrane made of genetically engineered naturally occurring molecules that make pores spontaneously. As the genome moves through the pore, an electric signal is generated showing how much current is running through it. Different nucleotides (the genome building blocks) give different signals which are decoded using special software, so reading the genome sequence.

Kary Mullis is another very interesting person whose scientific contribution has also been central to the postgenomic COVID-19 story. In 1993 he was awarded the Nobel Prize for inventing the polymerase chain reaction (PCR) when working at the Cetus Corporation, a biotechnology company in San Francisco.[7] The science journalist Nicholas Wade wrote in *The New York Times* in 1993 that biology now had two epochs, before and after PCR. Mullis was a badly behaved biochemist. He liked LSD. His private life was complicated. His Nobel Lecture describes the day he set up his first successful PCR with Fred, his technician. 'As he had learned all the biochemistry he knew directly from me, he wasn't certain whether or not to believe me when I informed him that we had just changed the rules in molecular biology.

"Okay, Doc, if you say so".' Mullis became notorious after leaving Cetus because of his scepticism that AIDS was caused by HIV. He was wrong about that, but he was right about PCR. PCR is a simple method for making with great speed many millions of copies of a DNA molecule. It works for SARS-Cov-2 but only after its RNA genome has first been converted into DNA using the enzyme reverse transcriptase, discovered by Howard Temin and David Baltimore (Nobel Prizes, 1975). Heating and cooling are essential steps in a PCR reaction. Using a heat-resistant enzyme to do the copying makes it much easier and much faster. *Taq* polymerase from the bacterium *Thermus aquaticus* is used. It came from hot springs in the Yellowstone Park, and grows best at 65–70°C. It is said that early in the COVID-19 pandemic, demand was so great that supplies of *taq* polymerase began to run short worldwide. PCR is the commonly used appellation for the test. Its full name is Rt-qPCR, Rt standing for reverse transcriptase, and q for quantitation, because the test result gives the amount of DNA it has found, an accurate measure of the amount of RNA on the nose/ throat swab.

Sydney Brenner's AD era goes back to Watson and Crick in 1953. Its twenty-first-century progeny, next generation genome sequencing, is utterly dependent on electronic computing, which in turn is utterly dependent on the transistor, much miniaturized. In 1956 John Bardeen, William Shockley and Walter Brattain were awarded the Nobel Prize for inventing it. The type that has taken over the world, the MOSFET (metal oxide semiconductor field effect transistor), was invented in 1959. And in the virologist's world, the 1950s was a very productive decade as well. Evidence produced almost simultaneously in 1956 by Heinz Fraenkel-Conrat in California and Gerhard Schramm in Germany showed that a virus genome could be made of RNA. It was not an animal virus, but one that infects tobacco plants, tobacco mosaic virus (TMV). TMV – called thus because infected tobacco plants have mottled leaves – was already very famous[8] because it was the first infectious agent to be categorized as something special, unusual and different from bacteria because of its distinctive properties in the laboratory (by Dmitri Ivanovsky in 1892), the first infectious agent to be called a virus (by Martinus Beijerinck in 1898), the first virus to be shown to be just a molecule (even it was a complex one), when it was crystallized by Wendell Stanley in 1935 (Nobel Prize, 1946), the first virus to be seen in the electron microscope (in 1939), the virus that officially drew Jim Watson to Cambridge in 1951 to work on its structure, the first virus to have its particle structure worked out accurately using X-ray crystallography (by Rosalind Franklin in 1955), and the first virus to be seen in the electron microscope by negative staining, the technique invented by Sydney Brenner and Bob Horne.

There are other interesting linkages as well, some important, and some inconsequential. Like Frederick Sanger, Bardeen was awarded two Nobel Prizes, though his were for Physics and Sanger's were for Chemistry. And both Bardeen and Crick worked on magnetic mines during the Second World War. Gerhard Schramm was a member of the Nazi Party and had been in the SS. He continued to do full-time fundamental biochemical work on TMV throughout the Second World War.

It is reasonable to speculate that because of Crick and Brenner's massive curiosity about the mechanisms that made living things work and their high gossip frequency that Lewis Carroll's description would be a good guess at what their discussions over 20 years might have sounded like:

'The time has come', the Walrus said,
'To talk of many things:
Of shoes – and ships – and sealing wax –
Of cabbages – and kings –
And why the sea is boiling hot –
And whether pigs have wings.'

While climate change worries in the 1950s and 1960s in Britain were about cooling, rather than warming and a *hot sea*,[9] Crick's father ran a boot and *shoe* factory and Brenner's was still mending leather *footwear* in his eighties. And Crick was useless at the traditional string-and-*sealing wax* approach to experimental science; he was very relieved when the apparatus he had built for his PhD project, which he had started just before the Second World War, had been destroyed when the physics department at UCL was blown up by a land mine during the London Blitz, so he didn't have to continue trying to measure the viscosity of water. But particularly important regarding COVID-19 was their interaction in Brenner's rooms at King's College Cambridge on Good Friday 1960[10] during discussions about a short-lived RNA that seemed to have something to do with gene expression. Suddenly they both realized that it was messenger RNA (mRNA). 'At this precise point, Francis and Sydney leapt to their feet. Both began to gesticulate. To argue at top speed in great agitation.

9

A red-faced Francis. A Sydney with bushy eyebrows. The two talked at once, all but shouting. Each trying to anticipate the other.' This simultaneous realization had an interesting pedigree. The foundational events were studies on radioactive RNA in virus-infected *E. coli* carried out at Oak Ridge by Elliot Volkin and Lazarus Astrachan in 1956, and the study called the PaJaMo (pronounced pyjama) experiment, carried out in the attics of the Pasteur Institute in Paris by Arthur Pardee, François Jacob and Jacques Monod on gene control in *E. coli*, published in 1959. The hunt for mRNA as a molecule started in earnest when Sydney Brenner and François Jacob went to Caltech and François Gros from the Pasteur Institute went to Harvard to use the special facilities in the American labs to look for it. At Caltech, Brenner and Jacob used amino acids made with heavy isotopes of carbon and nitrogen, using them to separate the protein synthesis machinery of a virus-infected *E. coli* by spinning in an ultracentrifuge and looking for newly made radioactive mRNA. After centrifuging, the plastic tubes had to be pierced with a needle and the liquid collected drop by drop. Many of the experiments failed. The final one was performed on the day John F. Kennedy was nominated for the presidential election. Brenner and Jacob joked that 'We're going to see if *we* receive a nomination now!' Their success was announced by Gros and Brenner at a symposium in 1961 sponsored by organizations including the US Public Health Service, the Rockefeller Foundation, the Atomic Energy Commission and the US Air Force.[11] Not only was this research of fundamental importance for understanding how life works, it filled a crucially important gap about messenger RNA described by Francis Crick as 'Is he in heaven? Is he in hell? That damned elusive Pimpernel.' He thought that the failure to find it earlier had been the one great howler in molecular biology: 'the only thing one is thankful for is that it wasn't all done by someone, as it were, outside the magic circle, because we would all have looked so silly.'[12] The magic circle of molecular biologists at this time can be identified as a brilliant example of a Ludwik Fleck thought-collective, a co-operative group practising provisional, raw and cautious science. Fleck was a Polish medical microbiologist who was a very important and creative sociologist of science as well as a developer of vaccines under the most difficult and frightful circumstances[13] – when he was a Jewish prisoner in Auschwitz and Buchenwald, where he produced 200,000 doses of a useless vaccine for the SS and 2,000 of a good product for fellow camp inmates, and for the Germans to test if they wondered why vaccinated soldiers fell ill.

Messenger RNA was used 60 years later as the crucially important component of successful COVID-19 vaccines, and the SARS-CoV-2 genome acts as messenger RNA at the beginning of an infection.

2

Coronaviruses:
The Beginning

We view COVID-19 through a postgenomic prism. The routine but gold-standard diagnostic PCR test made specific by WGS, the use of WGS to search for variants in real time, and the effective messenger RNA vaccines are all products of the Postgenomic Age. But a mature coronavirus science had already developed before its arrival. Electron microscopy was present at its birth. The first electron microscope that gave a better resolution than a light microscope was built in Berlin in 1933 by Ernst Ruska (Nobel Prize, 1986). Machines became commercially available in 1939. Ruska's father was Professor of the History of Science in Heidelberg and in Berlin, and his uncle Max was an astronomer. Ruska got his Doctorate when he was 28 and his Habilitation (an essential requirement for a licence to be a university teacher, based on a research thesis) ten years later. June Almeida's background and career were very different. Her father was a bus driver. She was brought up in a Glasgow tenement. The death from diphtheria of her young brother when she was 10 left a deep impression and stimulated an interest in science, at which she did well in school. But she had to leave at the age of 16 because no funds were available for her to continue her education. She became a hospital pathology laboratory technician in Glasgow, then had a similar job in London, and emigrated to Toronto with her husband. She took a post at the Ontario Cancer Institute as an electron microscope technician. She had ultra-green fingers, and soon her name began to appear as joint author on scientific papers. She developed a particular interest in classifying viruses according to the structure of their particles, paying particular attention to the nature of the spikes on their surface. In 1964 she was head-hunted by Professor Tony Waterson, newly appointed head of Medical Microbiology at St Thomas's Hospital Medical School in London, and she established herself in its basement with her new electron microscope.

Her reputation for pushing the virus visualization boundaries had spread, and in 1966 David Tyrrell, head of the Medical Research Council Common Cold Research Unit on Salisbury Plain, sent her human airway organ culture material infected with two viruses: 229E, isolated by the virologist Dorothy Hamre from the respiratory tracts of medical students at the Chicago School of Medicine, and B814, isolated from throat swabs and nasal washing from English boarding school pupils suffering from colds. June found virus particles resembling those of infectious bronchitis of chickens, first seen in the electron microscope by a group of scientists in Cambridge in 1964. Their surface was covered with a distinct layer of projections with a narrow stalk and a head. She had been the first to see human coronaviruses.

June had seen such particles before when studying the viruses that caused infectious bronchitis of chickens and mouse hepatitis. But her paper had been rejected. The referees said that her images were only bad pictures of influenza.[1]

A note in the world-leading scientific journal *Nature* in November 1968 announced the name 'coronavirus'. It said, 'In the opinion of ... eight virologists [they termed themselves "an informal group"] these viruses (avian infectious bronchitis, mouse hepatitis and human strains including B814 and 229E) are members of a previously unrecognised group which ... should be called the coronaviruses, to recall the characteristic appearance by which these viruses are identified in the electron microscope.' The fringe of petal-shaped projections recalled the solar corona. June's name headed the list of eight (though the list was in alphabetical order).

She formally retired in 1984, long before coronaviruses had achieved a reputation as being nothing more than trivial entities that caused colds and as viruses only of serious interest to veterinarians. By then, her reputation rested on her pioneer work on rubella and hepatitis B.[2] Among other signal achievements, her work on human wart virus in Canada was very highly regarded. The organ culture method used to grow human coronaviruses by David Tyrrell had impressed her a lot, and she used it at St Thomas's in an attempt to grow wart viruses. The organ was a bit of skin cut from my arm. I still have a scar to prove it. She had a wry sense of humour and I have little doubt that the naming after her in September 2020 of the new COVID-19 laboratory at Guy's Hospital would have caused amusement. The official history of St Thomas's opines that its disdainful dislike of and rivalry with Guy's, which came to a head when medical students from Guy's rioted in the St Thomas's operating theatre on 16 December 1836, has died down. As a St Thomas's person, I am not so sure. The emergence of SARS in 2002 transformed our appreciation of human coronaviruses. Until then, interest in them as causes of human infections had been small. The ones that caused the common cold were very difficult to grow, and the trivial nature of the illnesses they caused and the lack of any treatment meant that there was no incentive to develop a test. The Common Cold Research Unit closed in 1990. Studying respiratory viruses of that kind, looking for new ones, and researching their modes of spread had become unfashionable.

Well before the emergence of SARS the pathology of the brain complications seen in mouse hepatitis had stimulated studies looking for a possible coronavirus role in the causation of multiple sclerosis. The results were inconclusive, as were the investigations on whether coronaviruses caused diarrhoea in babies; porcine epidemic diarrhoea coronavirus caused acute diarrhoea and high mortality in new-born piglets. Nevertheless, coronaviruses still intrigued virologists. They have the largest genomes of all RNA viruses. Determining how they worked was an intellectual challenge worth responding to, whatever the veterinary or medical benefits. The research had early practical implications. Studies in the 1980s using the laborious and tedious sequencing methods of the day, involving the cloning in *E. coli* of DNA produced by reverse transcription of RNA from purified virus, showed that an apparently new coronavirus, porcine respiratory coronavirus, was in fact a variant of the pig gastroenteritis virus which had changed due to the loss of a chunk of sequence coding for the spike protein and the accumulation of multiple mutations in another virus gene.[3]

The basic information about how coronaviruses work that had accumulated over several decades has had immediate relevance to our understanding of SARS-CoV-2 infections at the molecular and cellular level. The virus genome is a long RNA molecule made of more than 30,000 building blocks, called nucleotides. There are four different nucleotides in an RNA molecule. Their arrangement along the genome molecule is its sequence. It acts as a messenger RNA coding for virus proteins when it gets into a cell, so their manufacture starts immediately after its entry. A complex and highly regulated process then begins. Big proteins are made which are cut into smaller functional ones by a virus enzyme, 3CL protease; some are enzymes that make more virus RNA, some subvert the host cells' synthetic machinery in favour of the virus, one proof-reads during RNA copying to get rid of possible mutations, and another helps to evade the immune response. Four proteins that make the virus particle are also made; newly synthesized RNA genomes become closely linked to the N (nucleocapsid) protein which then is surrounded by a membrane from the cell that has incorporated the M (membrane), E (envelope), and S (spike) proteins, forming the virus particle, which the cell then secretes. Molecular virologists were not surprised by any of these discoveries. The processing of big proteins into smaller ones by a 3CL protease was first demonstrated in 1968 with poliovirus. That discovery was made after complicated biochemistry experiments had been carried out using molecules labelled with radioactive isotopes.

Thanks to postgenomics and next generation sequencing similar discoveries about SARS-CoV-2 are being made a hundred times faster.

SARS

The first known case of SARS (severe acute respiratory syndrome) was documented on 16 November 2002.[4] The patient suffered from atypical pneumonia and lived in Foshan City, Guangdong Province, China. More people fell ill and the infection continued to spread, but China did not report the outbreak to the World Health Organization (WHO) until 11 February 2003, by which time there had been 300 cases and five deaths. A new strain of influenza was feared and on 20 February the WHO activated its Global Outbreak Alert and Response Network, and 11 laboratories in the WHO Global Influenza Surveillance Network began work. On 12 March the WHO issued a global alert on 'Cases of severe respiratory illness that may spread to hospital staff', and a second WHO alert was issued on 15 March; cases had occurred not only in China but in Hong Kong, Vietnam, Singapore and Canada. On 2 April there had been more than 2,000 cases worldwide. Influenza and other well-known causes of viral pneumonia were soon ruled out by the laboratory network. Coronavirus was seen in electron microscopy of tissue cultures infected with material from patients and a deep lung sample (bronchoalveolar lavage fluid, BALF) from a SARS case.[5] This wasn't right. Coronaviruses didn't cause pneumonia. But other tests confirmed the coronavirus results, and sequencing of chunks of the virus genome (but not its full length; next generation genome sequencing hadn't yet arrived) showed that it was a brand-new coronavirus. On 16 April the WHO laboratory network announced that this conclusion was definitive. On 20 April the Mayor of Beijing and the Chinese Minister of Health were sacked; both had downplayed SARS. On 28 April more than 5,000 cases had occurred worldwide. On 17 May the first Global Consultation on SARS was held. It concluded that the WHO control measures were supported by the evidence; early identification of cases and their isolation, vigorous contact tracing and management of close contacts, and the prompt reporting of symptoms by patients worked. On 8 May there had been more than 8,000 cumulative cases worldwide. And on 5 July the WHO declared the outbreak to have been contained. There had been 5,327 cases and 349 deaths in China and 2,769 cases and 425 deaths elsewhere, nearly all in countries close to China with the exception of Canada, which had 251 cases and forty-three deaths. There were no deaths in the US, which had twenty-seven cases, and none in the UK, which had four cases. Laboratory tests were not important; the WHO note on the status of diagnostic tests for SARS published on 2 June said that tests sensitive enough to be useful did not exist and that case definition rested on clinical presentation and chest X-rays.

The case fatality rate of SARS averaged about 15 per cent, being very low in the young (6.8 per cent in those younger than 60) and high in the elderly (55 per cent for those over the age of 60).[6] Most SARS cases developed symptoms, and sufferers did not become infectious until 7–8 days after symptoms appeared. Virus appeared in the faeces, but later than in the respiratory tract. Mathematical modelling[7] explained why SARS was successfully seen off as soon as it was. It had a relatively low R_o number (the number of second infections occurring after a contact with a single one) and a very low value for theta, the proportion of transmissions occurring before the appearance of symptoms. Such low values meant that isolating or quarantining sick symptomatic patients effectively stopped transmission. Even so, things were complicated statistically, because there was overdispersion, meaning that virus transmission did not occur in an evenly distributed way across a community. The majority of infected people did not spread the virus, but a minority infected many in one go – superspreader events (SSEs). These were not rare. A doctor from Guangzhou in China, who had been treating pneumonia patients, and who was ill, stayed at the Metropole Hotel in Hong Kong on 21 February 2003. Seven people staying on the same floor of the hotel got SARS. Their return to their home countries triggered seventy cases in Singapore, fifty-nine in Hanoi, sixteen in Toronto, and over a hundred in Hong Kong. A patient in Beijing was infected in hospital and went on to transmit her infection to her husband, sons, daughters and son-in-law and set up a chain of infections in healthcare workers and hospital visitors, the final number of cases totalling seventy-seven. In Hong Kong and Singapore, 71.1 per cent and 74.8 per cent of cases occurred in SSEs, numbers reminiscent of Pareto's 80/20 rule, derived by him from the distribution of income in Italy at the beginning of the twentieth century, when 80 per cent of the wealth was held by 20 per cent of the population.

SARS has gone. But coronaviruses that kill and specialize in superspreading have not.

MERS

The first human case of MERS (Middle East respiratory syndrome) fell ill in Saudi Arabia in June 2012. He had pneumonia. A virus was isolated in tissue culture, and a PCR test for coronaviruses was positive. Gene sequencing showed that it was a new coronavirus that had not been seen before. Its source was dromedary camels. Many of the camels are infected and have no symptoms. Ninety per cent of human cases have contracted their infections in Middle East countries, the great majority in Saudi Arabia. More than 2,000 cases have been diagnosed worldwide, two in the US and five in the UK. So far, only one big outbreak has occurred outside the Middle East. On 4 May 2015 a Korean man returned to Seoul, Korea, from Bahrain, where he ran a greenhouse business. He fell ill on 11 May and was admitted to the Pyeongtaek St. Mary's (PTSM) hospital with pneumonia on 15 May. He was transferred to a teaching hospital (Samsung Medical Centre, SMC) on 17 May and a MERS diagnosis was made on 20 May. During his two-day stay at the PTSM hospital, twenty-six patients were infected with MERS. Another person exposed at the PTSM developed pneumonia on 27 May, and he attended the emergency room at the SMC. His stay there for 59 hours with vigorous coughing and diarrhoea led to eighty-two confirmed infections. There were other superspreader events; 83 per cent of cases were due to five superspreaders. The outbreak lasted two months and there were 186 cases, eighty-two in hospital patients, sixty-three in visitors, fifteen in nurses, and eight in doctors.[8]

Are superspreader events caused by people who are more infectious or do they happen because of the setting in which they occur, or is it both? We still don't know for certain. Superspreading – technically called overdispersion – plays a very important role in COVID-19 (chapter 8). The unevenness of overdispersion is a very common biological phenomenon. In groups of individuals infected with intestinal worms, it is routine to find that severe clinical effects are restricted to 'wormy people', the 20 per cent of the community who carry 80 per cent of the whole worm population. A Royal Army Medical Corps entomologist, Alexander Peacock, counted lice on soldiers in the Western Front trenches in the First World War. They were important because they transmitted a new disease, trench fever, caused by a bacterium, *Bartonella quintana*. Paradoxically, it saved many lives because it was not lethal, but made its sufferers ill enough to be invalided home. J.R.R. Tolkien and A.A. Milne suffered from it. A very strong similarity with COVID-19 was that about 15 per cent of those with trench fever went on to develop a chronic illness with symptoms including exhaustion, fainting, headache, shortness of breath, pain, lassitude and palpitations. Peacock found that while 95 per cent of the soldiers were lousy, most had twenty lice or fewer, while 2.8 per cent had more than 350 on their trousers and shirts. The most famous example of a super-lousy person is Thomas Becket, Archbishop of Canterbury, murdered in his Cathedral in 1170. He wore a hair shirt, then an ordinary shirt, then a robe, then three woollen coats, then a surplice, and then, finally, a mantle. As his body grew cold, 'The vermin boiled over like water in a simmering cauldron.'

Postgenomic next generation sequencing has made it a straightforward job for virologists to construct genetic relatedness trees. They put SARS and MERS into the *Betacoronavirus* group along with many other coronaviruses, including two common cold viruses, and ones isolated from cows, antelopes, giraffes, horses, pigs, rats and bats. The *Alphacoronavirus* group includes two more common cold viruses, and viruses from cats, dogs and bats. *Gammacoronaviruses* have been isolated from birds and a beluga whale, and many bird species have yielded many different viruses belonging to the *Deltacoronavirus* group.[9] The authors of this study, most based in Hong Kong, concluded that warm-blooded flying vertebrates have been ideal sources of coronaviruses, their aerial habits helping their spread.

3
COVID-19: The Disease

The first step in a SARS-CoV-2 infection occurs when someone breathes in infectious virus particles and the spike protein (S) of the inhaled viruses sticks strongly and specifically to a protein, ACE2, on the surface of cells belonging to the victim. ACE2 (angiotensin-converting enzyme 2) plays an important role in regulating blood pressure, and occurs on many cells in many organs. After latching on to ACE2, enzymes in the human tissues cut S in two, activating it to fuse the membranous coat of the virus with the cell membrane, allowing the internal components of the virus to get into the cell and take over its machinery, which it subverts so that it becomes devoted to making more virus particles. A protein-cutting enzyme called TMPRSS2 is important. These events start in the nose, where cells expressing ACE2 are far more common than anywhere else in the respiratory system; such cells get progressively rarer the deeper down one goes (although getting more common again in the lungs, as does TMPRSS2), explaining why in many people the infection goes no further. ACE2-expressing cells in the nose are ciliated. The cilia are moving hair-like structures that sweep away rubbish. The secretory cells responsible for runny noses do not have ACE2. Breathing carries the virus that has grown in the nose down into the respiratory tract and the symptoms that may develop include a cough, a loss of smell or taste, a sore throat, a fever, fatigue and muscle pains. Some get diarrhoea. In about 80 per cent of those infected, the infection goes no further, and is dealt with success-fully by the immune response, but in the remaining 20 per cent, enough virus has travelled down into the lungs to infect type 2 pneumocytes. These cells line the lung alveoli, express a lot of ACE2 and TMPRSS2, and play vital roles in lung function and its recovery after damage. Infection of them with SARS-CoV-2 can cause them to release DAMPs (damage-associated molecular patterns) and other molecules, which alert the immune system and can trigger mechanisms leading to the suicide of surrounding cells in an attempt to curb the onward spread of infection. This response is usually successful despite its negative effect on lung function. But in those destined to die, the inflammatory response runs out of control, going into a feedback loop which, rather than protecting the lungs, becomes more and more destructive.

Chest X-rays, CAT scans, measurements of blood oxygen levels, brain scans, blood tests for clotting prob-lems, and kidney function tests give enormous amounts of information about these things. They show that after first attacking the lungs, the SARS-CoV-2 infection in the seriously ill then goes on to cause problems in other parts of the body. Finding out where the infectious virus is growing and what damage it is causing at the cellular level needs tissue samples. This is difficult in live patients. Taking lung or brain biopsies is nearly always unethical because their results are not helpful as guides for treatment and doing them is not free from danger. These things do not apply to the dead. But post-mortems are exceedingly unfashionable.[1] Long gone are the days of the mid-nineteenth-century Viennese pathologist, Carl Rokitansky, who personally did more than 30,000 post-mortems and consequentially made important discoveries about pneumonia and other lung infections before bacteriology had developed as a science. It could be said that he is now better remembered for the jest he made about three of his sons, a doctor and two singers: 'One heals, the others howl.' Far fewer COVID-19 post-mortems have been done so far than Rokitansky regularly did every year. A comprehensive review of post-mortems performed in the first 18 months of the pandemic[2] found that only 455 had been described in the scientific literature. A typical finding was DAD, diffuse alveolar damage, where the walls of the lung alveoli become covered with a kind of membrane made of dead cells, surfactant and proteins, and whose presence leads to an accumulation of liquid in the lungs. Thrombosis – blood clotting – appears to be universal, particularly in small arteries, but also in large ones. Damage to kidney tubules is very common, and in some individuals, virus messenger RNA was detected in brain, heart, kidney and liver tissues, indicating not only the presence of virus but that it was active in them at the time of death.[3] But being in the postgenomic era means that enormous amounts of information at the molecular level can be gathered from a single blood sample, and groups of scientists like COMBAT (COvid-19 Multi-omic Blood

Atlas Consortium) have joined to exploit all the molecular techniques of the day.

By far the most important risk factor for developing a severe and lethal SARS-CoV-2 infection is age (see chapter 7). Severe disease in children is rare and deaths are very rare.[4] A very uncommon condition in children has occurred after infection, sometimes weeks later, called the multisystem inflammatory system in children, MIS-C. Effects on most organs have been described, including the skin and the heart. Cases usually get better.

The linear relationship between age and the development of severe and lethal infections has no parallel in history. No therapeutically useful explanations have yet been published. An outstanding question is why children are spared. Only one infection comes close, typhus fever, caused by *Rickettsia prowazekii*. Although a bacterium, like a virus it can't grow outside human cells and like SARS-CoV-2 it does that in the cell cytoplasm. It grows in the cells that line small blood vessels. Some of the best clinical information of the pre-antibiotic era comes from a trial of new sulphonamides carried out in the Naples outbreak in 1943–4[5] when lice ran rampant, helped by a shortage of soap and the crowding of citizens who had taken refuge from air raids in deep underground shelters. The drugs didn't work, but the outbreak was ended by puffing DDT powder up sleeves and trousers and other places compatible with the maintenance of modesty; typhus in communities is spread by lice. In the outbreak, mortality rates rose steadily with age, from 1.5 per cent for children aged 9 or less, to 58 per cent for those older than 65. Once someone is infected with *Rickettsia prowazekii*, the infection persists for life, usually without causing symptoms, although relapses with mild symptoms are common enough to be eponymized as Brill–Zinsser disease (we will consider Hans Zinsser again at the end of this book). No evidence has yet emerged that human coronavirus infections lead to long-term persistence of the virus. Second infections with a genetically different virus from the first one (so not a relapse) have been well described, differentiating COVID-19 from measles, in which the robust life-long and very strong immunity after an infection may well be due to long-term virus persistence, not as infectious measles virus, but in a form that continues to stimulate anti-viral immunity.

Most people infected with COVID-19 recover; one-third have no symptoms at all, and about 81 per cent of those with symptoms only develop mild ones. Symptoms become severe in 14 per cent of cases; these include an acute shortness of breath, low blood oxygen levels, and X-ray/CAT scan lung abnormalities. In 5 per cent of cases, the lungs fail and the patient develops shock and multiorgan failure. In these patients the immune system has run out of control, and small blood vessels seize up because of abnormal blood clotting.

Other factors as well as age increase the likelihood that a patient will develop a severe illness. They include being male, and conditions that include chronic lung disease, heart disease, high blood pressure, diabetes, cancer and obesity. Being in the postgenomic era has meant that looking for additional genetic factors that might determine COVID-19 susceptibility and severity has become a straightforward exercise.[6] Although it is still work in progress, human genome-wide association studies have already identified gene clusters with variants that may increase susceptibility to the virus.

One cluster is at the genome locus 3p21.31, which arises from Neanderthal DNA and confers more than a twofold risk of death for individuals under 60. Risk variants at this locus are carried by more than 60 per cent of individuals with South Asian ancestry compared to 15 per cent with European ancestry. The locus contains gene *SLC6A20* that affects a sodium transporter molecule that interacts with ACE2, gene *CXCR6*, that recruits immunological memory cells in the respiratory system to combat pathogens, and gene *LZTFL1*, which controls EMT, the epithelial-mesenchymal cell response in the lungs which can be beneficial in a viral infection. The effects of individual human gene variants seem small, but the combination of their effects could be significant. Polygenic risk scores (PRS) have already been developed for COVID-19.

Although SARS-CoV-2 has only a handful of genes and a simple structure, it has multiple weak spots which are targets for antiviral drugs. Antibodies that bind to the virus particle spike stop it sticking to cells. The 3CL protease that cuts the big virus protein made in a cell at the start of its infection into smaller functional molecules is another target. An inhibitor of it, PF-07321332/ ritonavir (PAXLOVID), shows therapeutic promise, as do molecules that mimic the virus RNA building blocks, nucleosides, poisoning the ability of the virus to copy itself in an infected cell.

The treatment of severe infections with antibodies has a long history. A child in Berlin with diphtheria was given an antiserum made in a horse on Christmas night 1891. The antiserum treatment of bacterial pneumonia was widely used in the 1920s and 1930s. It saved some lives, but not many, and, given the ubiquity and effectiveness of antibiotics, is now only of interest to medical historians. At the beginning of October 2020, President Donald Trump was given REGEN-COV on compassionate grounds, a cocktail of two monoclonal antibodies that neutralize SARS-CoV-2 by binding to two different sites on the spike protein. A trial has shown that the cocktail, called Ronapreve in the UK, speeds the resolution of symptoms and reduces the risk of hospitalization and death. Monoclonal antibodies were first created by César Milstein and Georges Köhler at the Medical Research Council Laboratory of Molecular Biology in Cambridge in 1975 (Nobel Prize, shared in 1984). Their results were published quickly, allowing scientists worldwide to develop them further; no immediate medical applications were evident at the time. But a Prime Minister was furious. They should have been patented. Milstein viewed patents as best kept separate from scientific discovery and said: 'I was not unhappy. Margaret Thatcher was.'

The virologist and immunologist Nobel laureate Macfarlane Burnet suggested in 1953 that corticosteroids might be helpful in treating severe viral pneumonia. But sometimes they did damage, so their use was controversial. For COVID-19 the matter was settled by the results of the UK RECOVERY (Randomized Evaluation of COVID-19 Therapy) trial comparing the mortality of hospitalized patients receiving usual care or dexamethasone 6 mg once a day for up to 10 days.[7] Dexamethasone reduced deaths by one-third in patients on ventilators, by one-fifth in those receiving oxygen, but gave no benefits to patients not needing respiratory support, and could even have been harmful to some. Dexamethasone is cheap and has a well-understood safety profile. The trial showed that it prevented one death that otherwise would have occurred in a group of eight patients on ventilators, or in twenty-five patients receiving oxygen. The trial took 98 days, its preliminary results were announced on 16 June 2020 and were adopted into UK practice later that day.

Nucleoside analogues stop COVID-19 in two different ways. Remdesivir stops the virus making new RNA molecules. Molnupiravir gets built into newly synthesized RNA molecules and fosters the accumulation of mistakes, leading to an 'error catastrophe', the virus mutating itself to death.

COVID-19 patients who have been in intensive care may develop post-intensive care syndrome (PICS), in which many leave the ICU with physical impairments due to the drastic life-saving procedures they have undergone; some have impaired brain function and/or psychiatric problems. A significant minority who have not been treated in intensive care go on to develop long COVID, in which symptoms persist for 4 weeks or more.[8] These include fatigue, cognitive difficulties, shortness of breath, mood dysregulation, headaches, muscle pain and insomnia. Fatigue dominates. There is no evidence that any of the symptoms can be explained by the continued presence of the virus, although such investigations are very rare because obtaining tissue samples to look for the virus is problematic. Long COVID is more common after hospital admission for COVID-19, as it is in middle-aged white women, obese individuals, those with pre-existing asthma, and those with poor physical and mental health.

The overlap of symptoms with those of chronic fatigue syndrome (CSF/ME) is very strong. An independent working group on CSF/ME submitted a detailed report to the Chief Medical Officer of England in 2002. It recommended that research 'is urgently needed to elucidate the aetiology and pathogenesis of CSF/ME'. Hypotheses abound, but there has been no elucidation so far, indicating that it would be wise to be pessimistic regarding positive results coming soon from searches for simple straightforward mechanistic explanations for long COVID, including an explanation of the paradox that, while it disproportionately affects women, vulnerability to and mortality from infection is higher in men.

4
Origins:
December 2019–
January 2020

Clusters of patients with a pneumonia of unknown cause epidemiologically linked to the Huanan seafood and wet animal wholesale market in Wuhan, Hubei Province, China, were noticed in late December 2019. The market sold fish, shellfish and a variety of live wild animals including hedgehogs, badgers, snakes and turtledoves, as well as animal meat and carcases. The first patient had been admitted to hospital on 12 December. By the end of December, seven cases had been admitted to the Hubei Integrated Chinese and Western Medicine Hospital in Wuhan. On 31 December a team from the Chinese Center for Disease Control and Prevention started its investigations. The market was closed on 1 January. Not said publicly in so many words, but the big question was 'Had SARS returned?' Investigations followed two strands[1,2] first, the methods used in 1966 by June Almeida and David Tyrrell, namely growing the virus in cells from the human respiratory tract and electron microscopy; and second, next generation sequencing. Getting bronchoalveolar-lavage fluid (BALF) was the starting point. BALF is obtained by putting 100–200 ml of fluid down a bronchoscope into the lungs, then sucking it out. BALF from three Wuhan patients was negative for eighteen viruses and four bacteria by PCR using commercially available kits. Patient number one was a 49-year-old woman, a retailer in the seafood market. But something grew in the human airway epithelial cells, and coronaviruses were seen in the electron microscope. PCR for betacoronaviruses was positive. Next generation sequencing showed that the virus was a new coronavirus. It wasn't SARS; its closest relative was considered to be a bat virus, BatCov Ra TG33, with a 96 per cent sequence similarity, not close enough to be its immediate ancestor. The new coronavirus genome sequences from three positives had been worked out by 7 January, and on 10 January they were posted on GISAID, the Global Initiative on Sharing All Influenza Data database, enabling the immediate development of specific and accurate PCR tests worldwide.

Is there any good evidence that cases of COVID-19 had been in progress long enough that, if action had been taken earlier, the progress of the virus could have been nipped in the bud? None has been presented. Identifying the microbial cause in a case of pneumonia is often very difficult. It fails more often than not. BALF is not used routinely. It is unpleasant and potentially dangerous. Infections coming from food are common, but investigation of those caused by novel pathogens are not straightforward and take time, exemplified by the very big outbreak in Germany caused by the new hybrid *E. coli* O104 which started in early May 2011.[3] Hamburg was its epicentre. Cucumbers were wrongly identified as the source, but not before the Hamburg

Health Minister had gone public, with very bad effects on the Spanish cucumber industry. The true cause, contaminated fenugreek seeds imported from Egypt, was not determined until 10 June. There were 4,075 cases and 50 deaths.

In my view, the speed of response in Wuhan to the new pneumonias was almost certainly faster than it would have been if SARS-CoV-2 had emerged in Europe or the US. Its speed certainly does well in comparison with reactions to other novel pathogens in the US.

Legionnaires' disease, essentially a severe pneumonia, caused 221 cases with links to the Philadelphia State Convention of the American Legion at the Bellevue-Stratford Hotel from 21 to 24 July 1976. Twenty-four people died, a mortality rate of 16 per cent. But it took 6 months for the Centers for Disease Control and Prevention (CDC) in Atlanta, the world's biggest and best-funded public health laboratory organization, to discover its cause, a hitherto undescribed bacterium.[4]

AIDS had been characterized epidemiologically as something new by 1981, and the name came into use in 1982, but its causative virus, HIV, wasn't discovered until 1984.[5]

And West Nile virus (WNV) wasn't even new when it emerged for the first time in the US in 1999.[6] Contracted by mosquito bite, it had been discovered in Uganda in 1937. For many years it circulated in Africa, the Middle East, Russia and parts of Europe. Most infections were asymptomatic or quite mild. But by the mid-1990s the virus had changed. It caused a more severe disease. A new variant had emerged. On 23 August 1999 two cases of encephalitis were reported in the New York borough of Queens. Investigations identified a cluster of six cases. Some antibody tests gave a positive result for St Louis encephalitis virus (SLEV), another virus spread by mosquitoes which had been causing localized foci of infection in the US since 1933, and insecticide spraying started on 3 September. At the same time there was a massive die-off of crows in New York City. It was concluded that this mortality was linked to mass poisonings. On 7–9 September a cormorant, two Chilean flamingos and an Asian pheasant died at the Bronx Zoo. Viruses were isolated from their tissues and from a crow with encephalitis, and samples were sent to the CDC. On 23 September genome sequencing indicated a virus closely related to WNV, later confirmed to be very closely related to a strain of the new variant virus that had been isolated in Israel in 1998. It was found in the brains of patients who had died of encephalitis. The test results for St Louis encephalitis were not particularly specific but fitted the clinical diagnosis and so had been misleading, and the 'poisoning' of the crows was not a scientific conclusion but pure guesswork.

The US WNV discovery timeline in 1999 is uncannily similar to that of COVID-19 in Wuhan in 2019, in spite of the fundamental difference in the mode of transmission, mosquito bites rather than viruses in the air. Bearing in mind that institutions can forget,[7] it is interesting to note that the CDC's progenitor was MCWA, Malaria Control in War Areas, an organization set up in 1942, 6 months after the attack on Pearl Harbor, to research and control mosquito-borne infections. It became CDC in 1946. Other similarities between the WNV and SARS-Cov-2 abound. Both cause the severest infections in the elderly, in those with pre-existing health conditions, and in those suffering from socioeconomic deprivation. Both spread inexorably across North America, though WNV took longer; planes fly faster than mosquitoes. However, US citizens have been a lot luckier with WNV because only one out of every 140 infections causes severe infections, meningitis and encephalitis, and in the 20 years since its arrival, only 2,376 people have died from them. Several vaccine candidates for humans have been developed, but none have yet been licensed. WNV kills horses and several vaccines have been approved; the first was licensed for veterinary use in 2003.

Censorship is to be expected in countries with authoritarian governments, but it is not restricted to them. In the UK, bovine spongiform encephalopathy (BSE) had been identified as a new disease by the end of 1986. For the first 6 months of 1987, there was a policy of restricting information about it because of concern about 'the possible effects on exports and the political implications'. It was described as a policy of 'total suppression'. Official veterinarians were directed not to consult research institutes or university departments or publish anything about BSE or discuss it at meetings without clearance. Proposed publications about it were refused permission for their submission to the leading British veterinary journal.[8] In May 1987 there had been thirteen suspected and six confirmed cases in cattle. The total suppression policy was abandoned in October when case numbers had risen to 120 suspected and twenty-nine confirmed.

Where did SARS-CoV-2 come from? On 24 January 2020, my guess was that it was from an animal that had been infected with a bat coronavirus, with the changes that led to the species jump giving it the ability to infect humans.[9] No firm evidence to support or refute this hypothesis has yet emerged.

Was the Wuhan outbreak – which precipitated the pandemic – started by a leak from the Wuhan Institute of Virology or other laboratories in Wuhan? Transmission of nasty pathogens within and from laboratories has a long and tragic history. The Report of the Typhus Research Commission of the League of Red Cross Societies to Poland, which investigated the 1920 epidemic,[10] was dedicated to the memory of Conneff, Cornet, Jochman, Luthje, von Prowazek and Ricketts, 'who as a consequence of their researches contracted the disease and died'; and one of the authors of the report, Bacot, died from typhus contracted during his work in the year of its publication; and the 1951 account of the Rockefeller campaign against yellow fever[11] lists six of its scientists who died from it, Cross, Stokes, Noguchi, Young, Hayne and Lewis.

Establishing how a pathogen has escaped from a laboratory is often very difficult. Pessimism was in order that any kind of investigation run remotely by US spooks into events in Wuhan in 2019 could be definitive. Pessimism was correct. It wasn't. Difficulties are exemplified by the events in Birmingham, England, in August 1978, when Mrs Janet Parker, a medical photographer in the University Medical School, contracted smallpox. She never recovered, and became the last person to be fatally infected with smallpox in the world. The definitive diagnosis of her illness was made by electron microscopy. Work on smallpox was being carried out in the Medical Microbiology Department, but not in Mrs Parker's department, which was on a different floor from the smallpox lab. However, studies on the virus that had infected her showed beyond reasonable doubt that it was the same as one that was being studied downstairs at the time. A detailed investigation was carried out for the Government, involving observers from the World Health Organization and many experts. Its substantial report was published after a twelve-day trial which found the university not guilty of health and safety breaches after many witnesses had undergone rigorous cross-examination (with the exception of the Head of the Medical Microbiology Department who had committed suicide, dying on 6 September 1978), and detailed scientific tests of possible air-borne routes of transmission had been evaluated.[12] The report's foreword stated, 'The case against the University was dismissed. The way in which the outbreak of infection occurred remained unexplained.'

For a pathogen to escape from a laboratory, it has to be there in the first place. Sometimes investigating such an event is easy, at least to begin with. On 3 August 2007, cases of foot and mouth disease (FMDV) were diagnosed in southern England 6 km from Pirbright, the location of the only laboratory in the UK holding and handling the virus.[13] On the same site there was also an FMDV vaccine-manufacturing factory. Any doubts about the origin of the virus disappeared completely when genome sequencing showed that the outbreak strain was one that hadn't circulated anywhere in the world for years, had only existed in laboratories and vaccine plants, and was being handled in the labs and the vaccine factory at Pirbright just before the outbreak. Two official investigations were carried out and their reports were published a month after the outbreak. Waste from the vaccine factory containing live virus had escaped from the 40-year-old drains through which it was travelling to be disinfected, and then got onto the wheels of trucks leaving the site which were being used by workmen upgrading it (and renewing the drains).

If the SARS-CoV-2 virus escaped from a Wuhan laboratory to start the pandemic, how did it get there in the first place? Attention[14] has focused on the possibility that coronavirus gain-of-function experiments being performed there, particularly ones in which bat viruses were being altered genetically to see if they could grow better in human cells or mice. In theory such experiments could have created a virus like SARS-Cov-2, but the genetic differences between bat coronaviruses and SARS-CoV-2 are quite big, and many specific mutations in specific parts of any known bat virus genome would be needed for its creation, an event requiring an enormous amount of luck to be successful. A lot of bad luck would then be needed for this virus to escape. The likeliest route for this would be for a scientist in the lab to catch the virus, then pass it on person-to-person outside the lab. If the virus got into the drains, its dilution in the waste before it was disinfected, and the need to breathe some in, would make it very unlikely that such escaped virus could go on to infect anybody.

5
Fangcangs and Nightingales: February–April 2020

The World Health Organization declared a 'Public Health Emergency of International Concern' on 30 January 2020. By then there had been 7,735 COVID-19 cases in China diagnosed by PCR, and 170 deaths, and eighty-two PCR-positive cases had occurred outside China. It is certain that PCR positives fell far short of the actual number of infections. The virus had already spread to other countries in Asia and to Europe and North America. The pandemic was under way.

Wuhan was locked down on 23 January and a *cordon sanitaire* was imposed. This was two days before the start of the Chinese Lunar New Year National Holiday, when it was customary for people to travel home for the break. Virus spread continued. By 11 February there were 44,672 PCR-positive cases in China. More than 60 per cent were in Wuhan. At the beginning of February, hospital beds for COVID-19 patients were full there. On 5 February, three Wuhan exhibition centres and stadiums were converted into Fangcang shelter hospitals, with 4,000 beds. Thirteen more were opened by

22 February, providing a total of 13,000 beds.[1] Criteria for admission to a Fangcang shelter hospital were a positive PCR test, mild or moderate symptoms, no need for supplemental oxygen, an ability to walk and live independently, and an absence of severe chronic disease. Their prime function was quarantine, providing an alternative to home isolation for the infected, so protecting their family members. They also gave basic medical care and monitoring using basic lung function tests, and provided a degree of social support during isolation.

The Fangcang principle of setting up temporary hospitals during outbreaks of infectious diseases is not new. Joe Biden's great-great-great-grandfather ran the Ballina Union Workhouse in County Mayo from 1848 to 1850 during the Great Irish Famine, in which a major cause of death was typhus fever. Many died from it in the temporary fever hospital built against one of its walls. A particularly notorious example of a hospital hurriedly installed in premises built for another purpose is Scutari (on the Asian side of the Bosphorus in Istanbul), where Florence Nightingale worked in 1854 and 1855. The hospital had been built as an Ottoman barracks. It returned to military use after the Crimean War. Although set up as the destination for wounded soldiers who had survived transportation across the Black Sea, it became a hotbed of infection. Of British deaths in hospitals during the war, 16,334 died from infections and 1,724 from wounds.[2] Very similar to the thirteen new Fangcangs built in Wuhan was the 1,000-bed prefabricated hospital designed by Isambard Kingdom Brunel, without input from Nightingale. It is said that it was commissioned by a senior civil servant to show what could be achieved without her, that 'unforgivably bossy' and 'interfering' woman.[3] It had only just started working to full capacity when the Crimean War came to an end. It treated 1,500 men with a mortality of 3 per cent. The best example of the Fangcang principle in action in England before COVID-19 was the temporary smallpox hospital in Gloucester, South-west England, set up in a giant aircraft hangar at Brockworth aerodrome in June 1923. The smallpox was alastrim, a variant which had a mortality rate 30 times less than the classical virus. Alastrim took off in England in 1920. It had probably come from the US. The aerodrome hospital was needed because of the size of the Gloucestershire outbreak: 1,070 cases. The situation became so severe not only because Gloucester had been an antivaccination hot spot for many years, but also because during the outbreak deliberate misdiagnoses of smallpox as chickenpox were common. The motive was to evade isolation. The consequence was that smallpox cases remained in the community, spreading the virus.[4]

In 2020 the UK followed China in establishing its own Fangcangs, mostly in conference centres. In England they were called Nightingale Hospitals. The first, in London, opened on 3 April 2020. The Prime Minister, Boris Johnson, was admitted to St Thomas's Hospital with COVID-19 two days later. Irony abounds. St Thomas's had moved to its current location on the Albert Embankment opposite the Houses of Parliament in the early 1870s. Florence Nightingale had been consulted about its site. She was against it. She believed that its urban setting and the effluvia and dampness from the Thames would breed disease. She lost, fortunately for Boris.

Both the Fangcangs and the Nightingales had a short life. During the month of their active existence, the Fangcangs cared for about 12,000 patients. By 10 March, they were empty. The Nightingales were never used for patients with COVID-19, either for treatment or for isolation. Fangcangs and Nightingales were big. Appropriate comparators for size were the large twentieth-century tuberculosis (TB) sanatoria in Europe and America. They were very busy before the Second World War. In 1929 there were 22,500 beds in them in England and Wales, where Public Health Acts gave local authorities the power to compulsorily isolate patients with tuberculosis and give assistance to their dependants, powers that were hardly ever used.[5] Saranac Lake in the Adirondacks set the scene for TB sanatoria in the US. The tuberculosis analogue of the PCR test for COVID-19 used in the sanatoria was staining sputum for the tubercle bacillus. While not quite as sensitive, it gave results faster. It remains a mainstay of tuberculosis diagnosis today. The technique was introduced in 1882 after research in Berlin by Robert Koch (Nobel Prize, 1905) and Paul Ehrlich (Nobel Prize, 1908) and has changed little since. Some COVID-19 patients in Fangcang hospitals were treated with *quingfei paidutang*, a Chinese traditional medicine. It is a reasonable guess that it did as much good as the proximity of sanatoria to pine trees and the prescription in them of fresh air, cod-liver oil, exposure to sunlight, hydrotherapy (frequent baths) and zomotherapy (the consumption of raw meat). By far the biggest benefit from sanatoria came from the isolation in them of sputum-positive patients actively coughing and expelling thousands of tuberculosis bacilli which otherwise would have gone on to infect close contacts in the community.[6] Fangcangs did the same for SARS-Cov-2, as did the isolation facilities for London that were set up hurriedly in response to the occurrence of numerous malignant smallpox cases presaging a big epidemic in 1881, which was caused by a virus spread in a similar way to SARS-CoV-2: the smallpox hospital ships moored 17 miles down the Thames, the wooden three-decker *Atlas* and frigate *Endymion*, launched in the 1860s, and the twin-hulled former cross-channel paddle steamer *Castalia*. Vaccination had been made compulsory in 1853. Alone it wasn't enough, but when combined with case isolation, eradication of variola major in England followed at the beginning of the twentieth century. The smallpox ships were auctioned off at the Bull Hotel, Dartford, Kent, in December 1904 and broken up.

6

Test Test Test!
March 2020

'Test test test', said the World Health Organization Director General, Tedros Adhanom Ghebreyesus. His repetitive exhortation on 16 March 2020 affirms a basic aspect of the COVID-19 pandemic: the definition of a case in life and in death by the result of a PCR test. This postgenomic attribute makes it fundamentally different from all previous pandemics – influenza, cholera and plague – in which routine case finding and the construction of epidemiological statistics both during and after a pandemic were based on symptoms. The most frequently used pre-COVID-19 pandemic comparator is influenza in 1918–19. There was no test because the causative virus wasn't discovered until 1933. Until then a bacterium, *Haemophilus influenzae*, was thought by many experts, but not all, to be its cause. It wasn't found in some cases but occurred in others who were never ill. The enormous multi-volume medical microbiology text *System of Bacteriology* published in 1930 by the UK Medical Research Council put influenza into Volume 2, about bacteria. Its first chapter was by Alexander

Fleming, on staphylococci. Its preparation had obliged him to do research on staphylococcal variants. During this work he discovered penicillin. His colleagues at St Mary's called the book 'The Bible'; it was the last word on matters microbiological.[1] Today it is only of interest to antiquarian booksellers, even if it was correct when it said that vaccines against *Haemophilus influenzae* gave no protective immunity against influenza; large amounts of a vaccine had been made for the Ministry of Health for England and Wales and distributed in 1919 and 1920.

Neither were tests important in the second biggest influenza pandemic in the twentieth century, the 1957 Asian Flu. It emerged from China in February and arrived in England in July, peaking in September and October and again at the end of the year, killing 1,150 every week in England and Wales at its zenith. There were 81,000 excess deaths in the US. In its first wave in England and Wales more than half the deaths occurred in the under-55s. They tended to die quickly. Nearly 20 per cent perished before getting to hospital and two-thirds were dead within 48 hours of admission. Routine testing was never an issue because the tests of the day were so slow that by the time their results came through the patient was either better or dead.[2] Case definitions were based on symptoms. Cholera is the same. Test results do not drive the diagnosis or management of cases. Measuring the amount of watery diarrhoea passed through the hole in a cholera cot into a bucket below guides the amount of oral replacement fluid, which when properly formulated with salt and sugar reduces mortality fifty-fold,[3] a far bigger therapeutic benefit than anything yet devised for COVID-19.

Patients with COVID-19 shed the virus in their faeces. Unlike cholera, people haven't contracted it from sewage-contaminated water, as far as we know. But testing sewage, euphemistically called WWTP (waste water treatment plant) influent, by PCR has emerged as a useful way of monitoring SARS-Cov-2 virus levels in communities.[4] It uses the same principle as the Moore Swab, invented in 1948 by the Exeter Public Health bacteriologist Brendan Moore. His swab hangs on a piece of string in the sewer for 48 hours and traps microbes by filtration. For COVID-19, PCR has made sewage testing cheap and quick, but so far it has not achieved the pinpoint accuracy delivered by the Moore method for paratyphoid fever, which was first used to investigate repeated outbreaks of the disease that had occurred in North Devon in the 1940s. Moore tracked the causative organism up the sewers to the home of an ice cream van vendor, whose wife turned out to be a chronic carrier and the source of the organism.

Since the beginning of bacteriology at the end of the nineteenth century and the emergence of modern virology after the Second World War, tests have been used at the beginning of a pandemic to identify the causative microbe, and to try to spot the microbes that might cause one in the future. They have been used retrospectively as well. Genome sequencing in the twenty-first century of material from victims buried in Alaskan permafrost, preserved material from US soldiers, and samples from lungs kept in preservative in Berlin and Vienna has confirmed that all their owners, who had died in the 1918 pandemic with a clinical diagnosis of influenza, had indeed been infected with the virus, and sequencing of DNA from old bones and teeth has confirmed that the plague bacterium, *Yersinia pestis*, caused the Black Death. But never before 2020 and COVID-19 has a virus-specific test been so absolute every day in diagnosis, virus control measures, epidemiology and death certification. The gold-standard test is PCR, designed using the virus genome sequence. So COVID-19 is postgenomic; by the time the virus appeared, genome sequencing costs had fallen so low and its speed become so fast that sequencing its genome to identify it with precision and build a test using it was easy, and in principle rolling out and doing the test should have been almost as routine an exercise as a supermarket checkout operator scanning a bar code, which, like next generation sequencing, is another technology utterly dependent on MOSFETs and Nobel Prize-winning research, in its case the laser and the hologram.[5] The lateral flow test for SARS-CoV-2 also traces its founding principles to Nobel Prize-winning research, the development of partition chromatography by Archer Martin and Richard Synge at the Wool Industries Research Association Laboratories in Leeds in the early 1940s (Nobel Prize, 1952). The lateral flow test takes minutes and looks for the presence of the virus N (nucleocapsid) protein in a liquid sample. It is not as sensitive as a PCR test and it doesn't give any information about variants.

'If you've seen one pandemic, you've seen . . . one pandemic', says Adam Kucharski,[6] an expert on the spread of contagion. In other words, each and every pandemic is unique. SARS came close to causing one in 2002. It is sometimes said that its occurrence in Asian countries and the lessons they learned led to them being better prepared for COVID-19. But on balance it was harmful. Its biggest benefit was in its use as a metaphorical cudgel by Klaus Stohr, the WHO SARS research co-ordinator, to achieve an unparalleled degree of collaboration between virologists to identify it, which they did within a month. But the assumption was regularly made by public health policy makers that SARS-CoV-2 would be like SARS in being transmitted almost exclusively by patients with symptoms, including a fever, and that these clinical manifestations were very important indicators of infection. After all, both SARS and COVID-19 were novel genetically related coronaviruses from China that caused severe respiratory illnesses. In the first two months of the COVID-19 pandemic, testing in China concentrated on those with symptoms, and it was the same in the US and in Europe. But due to the application of PCR testing, it soon became evident that many SARS-CoV-2 patients presented with no symptoms. Despite the presence of the virus in the nose and throat, many individuals were asymptomatic, and those who developed them were infectious before their appearance. An early indication came from testing on a cruise liner. A passenger disembarked from the *Diamond Princess* moored off Yokohama on 5 February 2020 and returned to Hong Kong, where a PCR test was positive. The vessel was put under quarantine until 19 February. Most of the 3,711 passengers were aged 60 or over. Daily testing took place until 20 February, initially only on those with symptoms, but for the last 5 days was carried out on the asymptomatic as well. By then, 634 had tested positive, 306 with symptoms and 328 without.[7] By April 2020 the danger of relying on symptoms to identify cases, in particular those that might transmit infection, was becoming evident. An editorial published on 24 April 2020, in the influential *New England*

Journal of Medicine, was entitled 'Asymptomatic transmission, the Achilles heel of current strategies to control Covid-19'. It commented on a detailed investigation of a nursing home outbreak which showed that virus transmission by the asymptomatic was important. It was prescient. A review of COVID-19 outbreaks in care homes in Europe, North America, China, South Korea and Australia that had occurred in 2020 looked at reports from 8,502 care homes with 214,380 residents. There were 25,567 confirmed cases; 37 per cent were hospitalized, but 31 per cent had no symptoms.[8] And a definitive review of forty-three studies that had identified an infection by PCR on nasopharyngeal swabs and eighteen that identified a previous infection using antibody testing found that at least one-third of SARS-Cov-2 infections were asymptomatic.[9]

It was MERS, not SARS, that caused Korea to be far better prepared for COVID-19 than most other countries. The socioeconomic impact of the 2015 MERS outbreak was estimated to be US$8.5 billion. A paper published in 2018 endorsed by the Korean Society of Infectious Diseases[10] said that lessons learned included, 'The first line of defence is not the thermal scanner at the airport. It is doctors in the community clinics/hospitals, and 'Aggressive strategy for quarantine may be necessary, especially when large numbers of individuals are exposed in the health-care settings'.

7
The Epidemiologic Transition: Setting the Scene for COVID-19

By 2020 the scene had been set to maximize the impact of COVID-19. We had been in the Fourth Stage of the Epidemiologic Transition for years when the pandemic began. Epidemiologic Transition theory provides a convincing classification and staging of the major determinants of death throughout human history.[1,2] Its first stage was the *Age of Pestilence and Famine*. Life expectancy ranged from 20 to 40. Most of human history has been spent in this stage. Its second stage was the *Age of Receding Pandemics*, which for richer nations began in the middle of the nineteenth century. Separating human faeces from drinking water, and better diets, were crucial. Life expectancy rose from 35 to 50. The third stage, the *Age of Degenerative and Man-made Diseases,* had started by the 1920s, and made rapid progress after the Second World War. Isolation hospitals, vaccines, DDT and antibiotics hit the microbes and their methods of spread. Deaths from infectious diseases declined and were overtaken by those from other causes. A striking example of this change was shown by MMR – not the mumps, measles and rubella vaccine, but mass miniature radiography, which was used to detect lung tuberculosis. Its apotheosis was in Glasgow in April and May 1957, when, in just 5 weeks, 714,915 people were X-rayed. The publicity campaign was more vigorous than those recent ones for COVID-19 vaccinations in the UK. There was a campaign song, 'An X-ray for Me', and lottery-like draws for the X-rayed. Prizes were a washing machine, a television set, a refrigerator, a holiday in the Highlands, a bedroom suite and a car. Enamel badges given to the X-rayed were prized. They ran out. Additional supplies had to be rushed from England. Sputum from possible cases was tested for the bacterium; 523 were positive. Lung cancer was detected in 347 individuals.[3] After Glasgow, MMR screening for tuberculosis continued, but the number of TB cases detected fell quickly and the number of cases of lung cancer, mainly a man-made disease, increased rapidly. Most TB cases were cured. Most lung cancers were lethal. MMR population screening stopped in 1969.

A fourth stage of the transition, the *Age of Delayed Degenerative Diseases*, started in the early 1960s. It was unanticipated. Death rates from heart disease, cancer and stroke fell, not only in old people but in very old people; deaths from these causes were delayed. In the US, heart disease deaths declined by more than 25 per cent between 1968 and 1978. Declines of this kind happened not only in rich countries but worldwide. Personal experience illustrates why this has occurred, as well as its timing. I started smoking when a medical student to disguise the dissecting room smell, but gave up in the early 1980s, a time when tobacco use was becoming socially unacceptable, good news for my heart and lungs as well as for the population at large. But in May 2019, I had a non-ST-elevation myocardial infarction (NSTEMI), a heart attack without significant electrocardiogram changes. While I was lying on a cold X-ray translucent table in the cardiac catheterization laboratory 12 hours after hospital admission, stents were put into my left circumflex and right coronary arteries, and an angiotensin-converting enzyme (ACE) inhibitor was prescribed. ACE inhibitors were first marketed in 1981, and coronary artery stents were first used in 1986. I had joined the club of customers of cardiologists whose interventions we expect to postpone our combustion in the crematorium. But the likelihood of death if we catch a SARS-Cov-2 infection increases daily. The relationship between age and a lethal infection is stronger and more straightforward than for any other infectious agent. Without exception, the older you are the more likely you are to die from the infection, and the infection–fatality rate increase itself rises very steeply with age. The most recent Annual Report of the Registrar General of Births, Deaths and Marriages for Scotland typifies the statistics. It says that 77 per cent of those who died with COVID-19 were aged 75 or over and 43 per cent were aged 85 or over; 9 per cent were aged under 65 and there were no deaths under the age of 25. The infection–fatality risks during the first pandemic wave in New York City in spring 2020, when 21,447 confirmed and probable COVID-19 deaths occurred, were 0.00972 per cent for those under 25, 0.116 per cent for 25–44-year-olds, 0.939 per cent for 45–64-year-olds, 4.87 per cent for 65–74-year-olds, and 14.2 per cent for those 75 and older.

The Fourth Stage of the Epidemiologic Transition means that the old are getting older and older. In 1977 there were 151,110 care home residents aged 65 or over in England and Wales. The 2011 census counted 172,000 residents aged 85 or over. In the ten years to 2019 in Scotland there was a 20 per cent increase in people aged 65 and over. And globally the number of people living with dementia more than doubled from 1990 to 2016, mainly due to population ageing and population growth.[4]

Paradoxically, some medical advances that have increased life expectancy are also bad news if COVID-19 strikes, such as being successfully treated for blood cell cancers or having an organ transplant. But such conditions are uncommon, unlike another human condition whose frequency increase also took off during the Fourth Stage, one that ranks second only to age as a risk factor for COVID-19 severity and death. It is obesity. In the 1970s a third of Americans were overweight. By 2010 this had risen to 74 per cent.

In California the highest grade of obesity increased the risk of death from COVID-19 4.18-fold. The percentage of obese males in Britain doubled between 1993 and 2013, when 67.1 per cent were overweight.[5] A study on the impact of obesity during the first wave of COVID-19 in England used the medical records of 6.9 million people aged 20–99. It found a progressive increase linked to body mass index (BMI) in the risk of admission to hospital, to ICU and of death, the increase starting with individuals with a BMI of 23 kg/m^2, a BMI at the top of the 'healthy weight' range.[6] And in South America obesity is increasing faster than anywhere else in the world, with higher rates of increase in individuals with lower incomes and where the impact of SARS-Cov-2 has been particularly severe.[7] A worldwide study by economists[8] examining the relationship between national wealth and deaths from COVID-19 found that a 1 per cent increase in the population over the age of 70 was associated with a 0.8 per cent increase in deaths/ million, and a 1 per cent increase in obesity prevalence was associated with a 0.6 per cent increase in deaths/ million.

I was a junior hospital doctor at St Thomas's Hospital in 1962–3, just before the fourth stage had got under way in the UK, but when countries like India were still firmly in the third stage; life expectancy there in 1960 was 39.93. Today it is 68.8. If COVID-19 had emerged in 1962–3, its worldwide impact would have been very different from its effects today. Demography means that the number of elderly victims would have been far fewer. And there were far fewer fat people. Pneumonia would have been the diagnosis, but it is quite possible that a novel cause would not have been suspected, because the microbial cause of at least half of pneumonia cases is never established, a medical conclusion that does not prevent the completion of an acceptable death certificate, even today. There would have been little pressure in the early 1960s to investigate vigorously, particularly respiratory illnesses suffered by the elderly with dementia, many of whom in the UK were still resident in antiquated mental hospitals, in which the transmission of infection was almost impossible to prevent. The tragic events in 1984 at Stanley Royd Hospital in Yorkshire, which at that time had 830 patients, with more than a third aged 75 or older, and kitchens built in 1865, show that even in 1984 institutional infections affecting the elderly generated little interest.[9] The care home industry was in its infancy. If pneumonia cases had been studied in detail, success would have been unlikely even if a virus had been suspected, because SARS-Cov-2 does not grow in HeLa cells, the human cell line that would probably have been used to detect it by looking for visible cell damage, or in fertilized hen eggs, in which influenza virus grows extremely well. SARS-CoV-2 grows in African green monkey kidney cells, Vero cells, but these were not available in 1962–3. The virus grows in ferrets and gives them a fever for a few days but no other symptoms, and it infects cats, mink and hamsters. The likelihood that any of these animals would have been used experimentally to investigate a case of pneumonia in an elderly person is utterly remote. And none of the characteristic COVID-19 findings could have been made, such as the ground-glass appearance of the lungs on a CT scan, or 'happy hypoxia' when blood oxygen levels are much lower than the patient's breathing rate predicts, or D-dimer levels indicating an activation of blood clotting. This is because the first CT scan ever of a patient was carried out – on a prototype machine – in 1972, pulse oximetry to routinely measure blood oxygen levels was not introduced until 1981, and D-dimer measurements did not come in until the 1990s. There would not have been any pressure on intensive care units as they didn't exist. The first one, at St Thomas's, a pioneer in the UK, opened in 1966. It is quite likely that if SARS-CoV-2 had emerged in 1962–3, its main manifestation in the records would have been at best an unexplained increase in excess mortality ascribed to that common condition, pneumonia. It would not even have joined as a puzzle another mysterious condition, encephalitis lethargica, which caused an epidemic in 1917–26, first noticed in Vienna and France, then going on to affect about half a million people worldwide, killing a third of them and leading to a condition like Parkinson's disease in another third, because unlike COVID-19 it had very distinctive and characteristic clinical symptoms and signs. Its cause has never been established.

A prescient analysis published in 1998[10] was entitled 'Emerging infectious diseases: The Fifth stage of the epidemiologic transition?'. It noted that population ageing was sweeping across the globe, that 'the compromised immune system of the elderly makes them particularly vulnerable to infectious disease, especially pneumonia and influenza', and that the number of people living in healthcare facilities is increasing, which, though serving a critical need, 'promote the rapid spread of infectious disease' because their populations are compromised by age. COVID-19 has removed the question mark. Its pathological characteristic is pneumonia. Care homes have been one of its main targets. It has put us into the fifth stage of the Epidemiologic Transition, *The Re-emergence of Infectious Diseases.*

8

Outbreaks:
Learning in Real Time

Throughout the Fourth Stage of the Epidemiologic Transition, epidemiological information about acute respiratory infections did not come from testing but from the notification of deaths from influenza, bronchitis and pneumonia; insurance claims from populations off work because of illness; and absence records of children from school.[1] Test results were not important. Not so for postgenomic COVID-19. PCR testing on a grand scale has been revolutionary. Many outbreaks have been detected that would otherwise have passed without notice. It is likely that without PCR, none of those in universities and colleges in the US (in which 130,000 students had tested positive by September 2020) and in the UK (where 56,000 tested positive in 2020)[2] would have been noticed. This is unlike the mumps outbreaks that occurred just before COVID-19 at Harvard, Boston, Bristol, Oxford, Cambridge and Edinburgh Universities, as painful swellings of the salivary glands do not go unnoticed and testicular worries incentivize men to seek advice. PCR testing also revealed that

COVID-19 outbreaks in meat- and poultry-processing plants have been common. A survey in the US[3] found that by the end of April 2020, 115 plants had been affected, with 4,913 workers testing positive, and a mortality rate of 0.4 per cent.

Outbreaks are as important to epidemiologists as earthquakes are to seismologists. They give vital information about how infections spread, their incubation periods and their effects on different individuals. This information makes it much easier to design rational control measures. A classic example in England was hookworm disease caused by *Ankylostoma duodenale* in Cornish tin miners at the end of the nineteenth and beginning of the twentieth centuries. The adult worm is 10 mm long. It lives in the small intestine, attaching itself to the gut wall with its hooked teeth. Eggs come out in the faeces, and only hatch at temperatures above 16°C; the larvae start an infection by burrowing through the skin and entering the blood stream, then travelling to the lungs, moving up the windpipe, and wriggling down the oesophagus to the small intestine. An infected person loses 0.3 ml of blood per worm per day. *Ankylostoma* disease only occurs in the tropics and subtropics. The English climate is too cold. It currently affects about one billion inhabitants, mostly in sub-Saharan Africa and south-east Asia. There was an outbreak of anaemia among miners at the Dolcoath mine. It was initially attributed to impure air. An expert, J.S. Haldane, was called in by the Secretary of State for the Home Department (the Home Secretary).[4] The air was pure, but Haldane repeatedly found hookworm eggs in deposits of human faeces in the mine, and these were particularly common close to the deep Engine

Shaft, where the temperature was 26°C. Most of the 700 Dolcoath miners were infected, but only 10 per cent were ill enough to seek treatment at the Redruth Miners' Hospital, three miles from the mine. 'Bunches', small boil-like inflammatory lesions on knees and forearms, were very common. These were the sites of entry of worm larvae that had hatched in the wet faeces that contaminated the ladders used by the miners to travel up and down the mine. Cornish miners were peripatetic. Their skills were appreciated worldwide. One of them had brought *Ankylostoma* back home, most probably from India, was fit to work, but then initiated a superspreader event. The outbreak fizzled out at Dolcoath after the introduction of crapping buckets for the miners and the application of chloride of lime and potassium permanganate to the piles of faeces.

For COVID-19, big outbreaks early in the pandemic set the scene. The 2,500 cases associated with the international gathering of the Open Door Church in Mulhouse in France from 17 to 24 February, the 5,212 cases linked to the late February meeting of the Shincheonji Church in South Korea, and the PCR-confirmed infection by one symptomatic singer of more than half of the sixty-one attendees at a choir practice in Skagit County, Washington State in the US on 10 March[5] have demonstrated the facilitation of transmission by people close to each other singing indoors, and probably led to its consequential prohibition in many countries. The outbreak associated with a Zumba dance workshop in South Korea in late February and early March, and the seventy-seven cases after the St Patrick's Day celebrations on 17 March at the Redoubt Bar and Eatery at Matamata in New Zealand, where the participants were encouraged to get themselves 'Shamrocked', showed the importance of heavy breathing. Nightclubs in South Korea had reopened on 30 April but were closed again on 9 May because of infections; by 25 May, 246 confirmed cases had been linked to attendance at five clubs in Seoul.[6] All these outbreaks were superspreader events. These can set off a chain of outbreaks, like the multiple ones started by a mask-free socially undistanced but attendee temperature-checked wedding reception with fifty-five guests on 7 August 2020 at the Big Moose Inn at Millinocket in Maine in the US. A guest (who didn't develop symptoms until 8 August) infected twenty-seven others. One of them worked in a care home 100 miles away and went on to infect twenty-four residents (six died) and fourteen staff, and another guest who worked in a prison infected forty-eight prisoners and eighteen staff.[7]

The R value, crudely the average number of infections contracted from single infected individuals, has had lots of publicity. Its apparent simplicity masks its complexity; it is not usually measured directly but calculated making a number of assumptions. It is not a measure of the severity of an infectious disease or the rapidity of its spread through a population.[8] Superspreading reduces its utility significantly, because the evidence shows that while most people with COVID-19 do not transmit an infection, a minority do, in a big way. The dispersion parameter, k, gives the measure; for SARS-CoV-2 it is about 0.1, corresponding to 10 per cent of infected people causing 80 per cent of new infections. For pandemic influenza, k is about 1; 45 per cent of infected people cause 80 per cent of new infections. Mathematical modelling shows that for an infection with a low k value, limiting contacts during activities that bring together large numbers of people who would otherwise not routinely come into contact would be a much more effective control measure than limiting contacts between individuals who meet regularly and often, and without strangers.[9]

Large outbreaks on cruise liners should come as no surprise. Norovirus outbreaks on them have been occurring for years, and have now been joined by COVID-19, on the *Diamond Princess*, the *Grand Princess*, other vessels, and Nile river cruises. More surprising were outbreaks on aircraft carriers, the *Charles de Gaulle*, and the USS *Theodore Roosevelt*, which had many infections on board during its deployment to the Western Pacific in March and April 2020. In spite of social distancing and quarantining, 1,102 out of 4,985 crew, including the Captain, tested positive.[10]

Tragically, outbreaks in care homes were not a surprise. On 21 March 2020, the World Health Organization issued 'Infection prevention and control guidance for long-term care facilities in the context of COVID-19'. It said that people living in care homes 'are vulnerable populations who are at a higher risk for adverse outcome and for infection due to living in close proximity to others'. A review of events during the first nine months of 2020[11] was confirmatory; 45 per cent out of 8,502 care homes on four continents had outbreaks with case fatality rates of 23 per cent.

As an experiment of nature early in the pandemic, the *Diamond Princess* outbreak was particularly revelatory. Test results had already shown that asymptomatic infections were common. The isolation on board of a large number of passengers (2,666, 567 infected with fourteen deaths) and crew (1,045, 145 cases, no deaths), frequent testing, and good information about the movement of people on the vessel, its design, and air flows within it, provided an excellent opportunity to assess the relative importance of transmission of infection by respiratory droplets that fall to the ground and don't travel far, aerosols that can travel further on the air, and fomites transfer via inanimate objects and surfaces. Aerosol transmission emerged as the most important, with fomites the least.[12]

9
Whole Genome Sequencing

Alvin Weinberg was worried that Big Science's domi-
nance would damage science overall. But he was a
physicist. Biology thrives on Big Data. It is a fundamental
characteristic of the Postgenomic Age. An outstanding
example is the work of the Wellcome Sanger Institute,
at Hinxton Hall, near Cambridge in England. Set up in
1992 to play a major role in the Human Genome Project,
and now a UK centre for SARS-Cov-2 sequencing, it is
one of the largest sequencing centres in the world. In its
25-year existence it has sequenced 18 quadrillion DNA
bases. Thanks to the massive impact of next generation sequencing, one-third of them have been delivered
in the most recent year for which data are available, a
rate equivalent to one human genome sequence every
3.5 minutes. It came of age thanks to the technical
developments that characterize the Postgenomic Age.
It played a key role in the first real-time use of whole
genome sequencing (WGS) to investigate an outbreak of
infection. In 2011 there was an outbreak of methicillin-
resistant *Staphylococcus aureus* (MRSA) at the mother

and baby hospital in Cambridge. WGS showed that the outbreak was significantly bigger than identified by methods that were state-of-the-art at the time, and that it had started 6 months earlier than had been thought. It also identified hitherto unsuspected links between mothers and between infants and mothers and mothers and their partners, and identified a staff member carrying the outbreak MRSA strain linked to its reappearance after an infection-free gap of 64 days.[1]

MRSA and SARS-CoV-2 are very different microbes. But WGS showed its utility early in the pandemic in England, also at a hospital in Cambridge and also in investigations of healthcare-associated infections.[2] A combination of genome sequencing and epidemiology identified many clusters of COVID-19 cases at the hospital in March and April 2020, with this information indicating virus transmission in twelve wards, nine of which had no known COVID-19 patients at the onset of the clusters. Six patients on out-patient renal dialysis were infected with exactly the same virus; the transmission route could not be established with certainty; some might have contracted the virus while being dialysed close to others in the open room where dialysis was carried out, or in the shared transport to the unit. They did not catch it in the renal ward, which also had a COVID-19 outbreak and which shared patients with the out-patient unit; the dialysis unit genomes and the renal ward genomes were significantly different.

WGS is not expensive once its infrastructure is in place. Compared with traditional fingerprinting methods for microbes, it is faster, more accurate, more reproducible and much more discriminatory. It can easily be performed on virus nucleic acid left over from a PCR test. In near real time it generates the information needed to characterize a microbe by the mutations in its genome in order to find out where it has come from, track its onward spread, and look for the mutations that might affect its ability to spread, its virulence, and the efficacy of vaccines, as well as giving information that can be used to work out evolutionary histories. It generates a massive amount of information which would be virtually useless without systems to analyse it and share it internationally. Acronyms abound. PANGOLIN (Phylogenetic Assignment of Named Global Outbreak Lineages) is one software tool. It was released on 30 April 2020. It assigns viruses to PANGO lineages – groups of viruses with very similar genome sequences – whose transmission, travels and fate can then be followed using packages such as CIVET (Cluster Investigation and Virus Epidemiology), which combines WGS and epidemiological information. Open access to information comes through GISAID, the Global Initiative on Sharing All Influenza Data. In the UK this work is carried out through COG-UK, the COVID-19 Genomics consortium; sequences are put on MRC CLIMB-COVID, the Medical Research Council Cloud Infrastructure for Microbial Bioinformatics. COG-UK was set up in April 2020. In its first year it sequenced more than 450,000 SARS-CoV-2 genomes.

The SARS-CoV-2 mutation rate is less than for most other viruses with an RNA genome. Unlike them, coronaviruses code for an enzyme that proof-reads when copies of their RNAs are being made in an infected cell, the point in the virus growth cycle when mutants are generated. However, enough of them survive to give WGS real fingerprinting power. By July 2020,

13,428 SARS-CoV-2 variants had been found, half of them having an effect on the protein that they code for.[3]

WGS on 26,181 UK virus genomes from the first pandemic wave, which peaked in April 2020 and which by June had accounted for 40,453 nationally notified COVID-19 deaths, enabled the identification of 1,179 transmission lineages, of which 33 per cent came from travellers returning from Spain, 29 per cent from France, 12 per cent from Italy, and 26 per cent from elsewhere. London and some surrounding commuter counties had the most lineages; rural Aberdeenshire in Scotland had one of the fewest. The rate of importation peaked in mid-March, when about 200,000 international travellers were arriving in the UK every day. After lockdown, on 23 March, many lineages fizzled out; the biggest ones with many members survived best. Many (1,650) genome types were found only once. They didn't move on to become transmission lineages, and died out.[4] A detailed WGS and epidemiological study in Scotland at the beginning of the pandemic showed how quickly the virus moved into the community after its importation. Ninety early introductions were linked epidemiologically to travel in Europe, seven to Caribbean cruises, and seven to travel to the rest of the world. A Chinese lineage was introduced at least ten times, but the majority of its introductions had come from Spain. The first confirmed case in Scotland without a travel history tested positive on 2 March, and a cluster of more than sixty cases without a travel history but caused by genetically related viruses occurred in Glasgow and Edinburgh between 13 and 31 March. A fourteen-case care home outbreak with no travel links broke out in Glasgow in mid- and late March.[5] WGS data, coupled with information about domestic and international travel, showed a similar pattern in the US, where by mid-March the risk of introduction of the virus by domestic air travel had begun to exceed that by international travel.[6] WGS has also given important information about localized virus outbreaks. Recommendations were made during the first wave of the pandemic that the best way to protect care home residents was to regularly test all who went into them to prevent the ingress of the virus.[7] A review of WGS data confirmed the importance and practicality of this measure. Outbreaks were most commonly due to single or few introductions, rather than a series of seeding events from the community, and studies showed that once the virus had entered, it persisted, despite extensive prevention and control measures being in place; that residents and staff were usually infected with the same virus; and that there was evidence suggesting that transmission between different establishments by shared staff might have happened.[8]

At Cambridge University between October and December 2020, 972 SARS-Cov-2 infections occurred in students and staff. Analysis of 482 genomes found twenty-three PANGO lineages. Most were introductions from outside that did not go on to form clusters of cases. One did. The likeliest starting point for its spread in the university was a group of ten students who had visited a nightclub. It went on to affect most colleges, as well as students taking twenty-eight different courses and 208 households in university accommodation. There was little spread into the community with the exception of some transmission to healthcare workers from medical students.[9]

New Zealand's remoteness and long-established effective border controls have given it a marked degree of protection from COVID-19. Its application of managed quarantine for all coming into the country, frequent PCR testing, extensive use of WGS, and high-quality public health system had made the country a very useful source of information about the virus. In its first COVID-19 wave between 26 February and 1 July 2020, 1,178 cases were diagnosed by PCR. WGS was carried out on 649 of them. Results show how it generated information about the habits of the virus that is useful to public health, and also indicated a weakness in its international implementation. During the first wave, WGS results showed that the virus was brought into the country by 277 people. Most (57 per cent) did not infect anybody, 24 per cent infected only one other, while 19 per cent went on to cause an outbreak. The biggest was a wedding where there was a superspreader event with ninety-eight cases that was caused by virus brought in from the US; traditional epidemiological investigations failed to spot five cases, which were only identified by WGS. Tracking the cases during the outbreak showed the effectiveness of the New Zealand strict lockdown, which started on 26 March, when the outbreak was in full progress with an R value of 7, meaning that on average each case was infecting seven others. Within a week it had fallen to 0.2.[10] By June 2020 community transmission of the virus had stopped in New Zealand. One hundred days later, on 11 August, four new cases were diagnosed. Their origin was unknown. An outbreak started, leading eventually to 175 more cases. WGS indicated a single source for the outbreak, but was unable to link the genome sequence to any close relatives in the international database. The best that could be done was to conclude that the virus might be related to one from South Africa, or England, or Switzerland. This investigation highlighted two issues, the patchiness of genome sequencing across the world, and the build-up of genomic diversity over time. By the end of 2020, the UK had had about 4 per cent of world COVID-19 cases, with its national genome sequencing comprising 44 per cent of the global dataset; for India it was 11 per cent of world cases and 1 per cent of the dataset.

Investigating the spread of infection on aircraft is difficult, because passengers disperse after landing. In New Zealand, however, arrivals were obliged to undergo managed isolation and quarantine for 14 days with mandatory testing for SARS-Cov-2. Sometimes evidence obtained this way showed clearly that passengers had been infected before departure and did not catch the virus during the flight. Twelve passengers tested positive on arriving on the same flight from India. The genomes fell into four lineages and there were more additional mutations in the group than had been observed in New Zealand during the whole of the first wave.[11] Some investigations were much more straightforward. A flight from Dubai arrived on 29 September 2020. Seven passengers tested positive in quarantine. Six had been infected with a virus with an identical sequence and one with a virus with a nearly identical genome. Incubation periods indicated that two of them, from Switzerland, were infectious during the flight and had passed the virus to four others, who were sitting in aisle seats not further than four rows away. The final infected passenger was a travel companion of one of the six, who stayed in the same room at the isolation and quarantine facility, and had caught the virus there. Five of the passengers, including the ones from Switzerland who had tested negative about 72 hours before boarding in Dubai, wore masks and gloves during the flight.

The power and utility of WGS in outbreak investigation and the rapidity and ease of spread of the virus were dramatically demonstrated in the state of Victoria in Australia during its second wave of infection. After some importations of the virus early in the pandemic, on 20 March 2020 the Australian border was closed except for residents returning to the country, who were obliged to complete at least 14 days of quarantine in a hotel or similar supervised facility. By the beginning of May the virus was virtually eliminated in Victoria apart from a meat plant outbreak whose source was never found. At the beginning of June, a surge in case numbers began. It started with a few cases in staff at a quarantine hotel, but then took off in the community. WGS showed that the origin of the virus was a family from Bangladesh who had stayed at the quarantine hotel. Case numbers increased rapidly, peaking in late August. International arrivals into Victoria stopped on 30 June, interstate travel in Australia was restricted, and local and state-wide lockdowns were introduced. Case numbers fell; the last was on 29 October. Between June and October, 10,426 cases were diagnosed in Victoria. WGS showed that 98.4 per cent were derived from the quarantine hotel event.[12]

10

Variants

Mutations are mistakes. Most of them are harmful to the virus and make it non-viable. They occur when errors are made during the copying of its nucleic acid genome, errors that are more common with RNA viruses than for those with DNA genomes. The bigger the RNA genome, the greater the number of mistakes: SARS-CoV-2 has a very large RNA genome, and gets by because it has a proof-reading enzyme (an exonuclease, colloquially called ExoN) that corrects copying errors and reduces the measurable mutation rate twenty-fold – but not to zero; it misses about 6 per cent of mutations. WGS results indicate that SARS-CoV-2 evolves at a rate of 0.3 non-lethal mutations every virus generation. There have been millions of such virus generations since the start of the pandemic, explaining why thousands of mutations have been detected. The value of most of them to investigators is to use them as labels to characterize the lineages and clusters used to monitor the spread of infection. Lineages of closely related viruses are quite stable in that they only accumulate about one or two mutations every month. Attention focuses on the lineages that have become very common, because their abundance raises the question that this may have happened because, in evolutionary terms, they have a selective advantage. Research has concentrated on mutations in the virus spike protein, which is essential for the virus at the beginning of an infection because it sticks to cells and then gets the innards of the virus into them, but is also its biggest weak spot as it is the main target for the immune response.[1]

By the time you read this chapter it will be out of date, maybe in an important way from the public health point of view, maybe not.

D614G was the first important spike variant to take off. It has a mutation at amino acid position 614 of the spike protein. Arising in Italy and called lineage B.1, from March 2020 onwards it spread worldwide, becoming common in Europe and America, and appearing in Australia. Laboratory research[2] showed that it grows better in human bronchial and nasal airway epithelial cell cultures and in hamsters and ferrets, and that the variant spike protein binds more effectively to the angiotensin-converting enzyme 2 (ACE2), the molecule on the cell surface to which the virus has to stick before getting inside to start the infectious process. It transmits 10–20 per cent better than the original Wuhan virus.

Lineage *B.1.177* has a mutation at spike protein position 222 and two others in different parts of the virus genome. The part of the spike protein affected by the mutation is not involved in sticking to ACE2. *B.1.177* was first detected in Spain on 20 June 2020 and was first found in the UK on 18 July. By the end of the month, it had been detected in Switzerland, Ireland, Belgium and

Norway, and by the end of August it had spread across Europe. After its introduction into the UK, it spread rapidly, the proportion of positive test results with it in England rising from 25 per cent at the beginning of September to 65 per cent at the end of October. Its expansion relative to B.1 went on until January 2021.[3]

On 20 September 2020 a virus sample was collected in Kent, in southern England. This was the first appearance of lineage *B.1.1.7*. Called the Alpha variant by the WHO, it had fourteen mutations that affected the proteins of the virus. Individually many of them had been observed before, but never in such a combination. Several affected the spike protein, including a mutation that caused an amino acid change at position 501, which increases the ability of the virus to stick to ACE2 and be more infectious and virulent in a mouse model. Some mutations are called deletions, because they lead to amino acids going missing from the protein coded for by the RNA in which they occur. Two amino acids at spike positions 69–70 had gone in *B.1.1.7*. This deletion might help the virus to evade the immune response. The second wave in the UK from December 2020 to February 2021 was almost exclusively driven by *B.1.1.7*. Other lineages also lurked in the UK. They had a spike mutation at position 484, which reduces the rate of virus neutralization by antibodies generated by a previous infection. This mutation was sometimes found in *B.1.1.7* viruses. But it did not seem to enhance their growth, another example of the general principle that how a virus behaves depends on interactions between all its genes. A third UK lockdown started on 4 January 2021. The daily number of positive PCR tests fell from 72,090 on 29 December to 2,500 at the beginning of

April, when 99.1 per cent of genomes sequenced were
B.1.1.7.

B.1.617.2 was detected during a surge in COVID-19
cases in India in December 2020. Called the Delta variant by the WHO, it has many mutations that affect the
spike protein. It does not have the spike 484 mutation,
but a very important one is P681R, which transforms a
proline amino acid in the spike to arginine.[4] For the virus
to successfully infect a cell, the spike has first to stick to
ACE2, then be cut twice to activate its S2 subunit, which
fuses the cell and virus membranes. P681R makes this
process more efficient by helping the first cutting step to
happen before virus particles leave the cell in which they
are growing, rather than waiting for it to happen after S
has stuck to ACE2. It was first found in England in March
2021. There had been a large number of introductions
from India. The number of cases grew rapidly owing to
onward transmission and large local clusters of cases, a
growth about 37 per cent greater than *B.1.1.7*. This was
due to the large number of introductions over a short
time, epidemiological factors specific to the communities
where it spread most quickly, greater transmissibility of
the variant itself, and, possibly, to enhancement of its
ability to escape the protection that comes from specific
anti-virus antibodies.[5] A very detailed study of an outbreak in China[6] showed that infected individuals made
much more virus and made it earlier after infection than
before. *B.1.617.2* went on to dominate the COVID-19
scene worldwide, and displaced the Alpha variant globally. Its increased transmissibility increased the leakiness
of the stringent border controls operated by countries
such as New Zealand, and significantly assisted the virus
to spread after a leak.

Then came variant *B.1.1.529*, PANGO lineage BA.1, first reported to the international genomic database GISAID by South Africa on 23 November 2021. Designated Omicron by the WHO, it has fifty-one mutations across the entire genome, with an unprecedented thirty-three in the spike protein gene, six of which had never been seen before, and twenty-five in the regions of the spike which are the main targets for neutralizing antibodies. It spread rapidly across the world. Attempts to control its international spread by travel restrictions were unsuccessful. In Scotland it caused superspreader outbreaks on 20 and 22 November. Case numbers then increased very rapidly. It outcompeted Delta. By 5 January 2022, the prevalence of Omicron in Scotland had increased to 91.1 per cent. Clinical data and laboratory studies showed that the prediction made from genome sequencing that it would be more successful than previous variants at evading immunity conferred by vaccination or a previous COVID-19 infection were correct.[7] It showed its ability as a superspreader at an office party in Oslo on 26 November attended by someone who had returned from South Africa two days before; eighty-one of the 117 attendees were infected, of which seventy-nine (98 per cent) had been fully vaccinated.[8] But sequencing information had not predicted that it would be more transmissible. Neither had it indicated that it would be less virulent, which it is. Laboratory studies have shown that its spike protein binds better to the ACE2 receptor than any other variant, and unlike them, is much less reliant on using the TMPRSS2 enzyme to get into cells. It can use other cell enzymes, cathepsin proteases, instead. These properties help it to grow much better in the nose because ACE2 cells with cathepsins are far more common there than ones with TMPRSS2. Its less efficient use of TMPRSS2 also explains the decrease in severity of disease. After infecting a sheet of Vero tissue culture cells engineered to express ACE2 and TMPRSS2 (VAT cells), the virus spreads from cell to cell, killing them and forming plaques, holes in the sheet. Delta plaques are much bigger than those formed by Omicron.[9] Although Delta plaques are laboratory demonstration distant from the events in the lungs of a patient, from the COVID-2 point of view VAT cells mimic those deep in the lungs, and the plaque size difference is very strong evidence that Omicron is significantly less virulent than Delta.

I started my virological career working on virulence in Newcastle disease, a chicken infection. Mortality rates caused by different variants range from nearly 100 per cent (when it first appeared in Indonesia and Newcastle, England, in 1926) to zero. Many infections are asymptomatic. There is a very strong correlation between virulence and plaque-forming ability.[10] It is often said that as viruses evolve, it is likely that they will get less virulent. Newcastle disease virus did. But the canonical example is myxomatosis, the rabbit equivalent of smallpox, deliberately introduced into Australia in 1950. Initially it killed more than 99 per cent of animals in under a fortnight; after two to three years the mortality rate had fallen to 90 per cent with sick rabbits surviving on average three weeks or longer. The Australian virologist Frank Fenner is remembered for two things: this myxomatosis research, and his small-pox eradication activities. His concluding remarks at a symposium on Newcastle disease virus in 1963 still apply: 'Natural selection works upon transmissibility, not upon antigenic structure or virulence as such. It affects either or both of these only insofar as they affect transmissibility.'[11]

11

Vaccines

The first detailed investigation into immunity after a coronavirus infection was carried out in the late 1980s on volunteers at the Common Cold Research Unit at Salisbury. They were infected with the common cold coronavirus 229E, and followed up a year later. Antibody levels had fallen, to zero for some, and six out of nine could be reinfected, although only one developed symptoms.[1] Vaccine-induced immunity is quite often inferior to that which follows a natural infection, so optimism was guarded about the protective effect from possible SARS-CoV-2 vaccines. History tells many cautionary tales about vaccine efficacy. The best model regarding protection against a respiratory virus by vaccination was influenza. Vaccines made in the traditional way, in which the virus is grown in eggs and then inactivated, give 60 per cent protection against infection to about 60 per cent of those who have been vaccinated. So the willingness of governments to make major investments in new products that might turn out to be at best feeble was a very big gamble. But some vaccinologists had a flying start, from MERS. Unlike SARS, whose spillover from its animal source was almost certainly a one-off incident with a very low probability of a repeat, MERS still flourishes in its animal reservoir, the dromedary camel, and transmission to humans will continue unless something is done. This stimulated research into MERS vaccine development, appropriately described by one research group after their success as 'a proof of concept for the prototype pathogen approach to pandemic preparedness'.[2] Research has concentrated on the virus spike, S, because antibodies against it neutralize the virus, for all practical purposes killing it. S works by using part of its molecule, the receptor binding domain, S_1, to stick to a particular protein on cell surfaces, the ACE2 receptor. In a two-step process, it is then cut by protease enzymes, changing its shape and activating another part of the molecule, S_2, which fuses the virus with the cell membrane, allowing its contents to get into the cell and start the infectious process. MERS vaccine developers had one goal, which was to get the genetic information coding for S into human or camel cells which would then manufacture it and safely stimulate an effective immune response. They used two very different ways to do this. Ten years before COVID-19 appeared, Oxford had developed a genetically engineered chimpanzee adenovirus that cannot grow in humans, ChAdOx1, to act as a vaccine vector to carry DNA sequences into cells to make a protein against which immunity is sought. In their MERS project, the researchers engineered a linkage of the tissue plasminogen activator leader sequence, already known to boost the immunogenicity of other viral proteins, to the S sequence. Trials in mice and humans of the vector with the modified MERS S sequence showed that it stimulated an immune response and protected animals against MERS.[3]

The AstraZeneca vaccine uses the SARS-Cov-2 S sequence modified in exactly the same way. US researchers used a different approach. They studied the structure of the MERS S protein in great detail and found that two amino acid changes to its structure made it resistant to being cut and made it more immunogenic. The messenger RNA (mRNA) coding for this engineered protein was incorporated into tiny lipid nanoparticles which protect the mRNA from destruction by enzymes which chew up RNAs, and transport it into cells to make the modified S. In experiments on mice, the nanoparticles stimulated the production of high levels of neutralizing antibodies and protected transgenic mice against lethal doses of MERS. Within 24 hours of the release of the SARS-CoV-2 genome sequence, on 10 January 2020, the US team had made mutated S, and 4 days later started to make S mRNA. Human trials began 66 days after the release of the genome sequence. Pfizer–BioNTech and Moderna vaccines followed. Within 24 hours of the genome sequence release, the Oxford team had started to design their modified S, and started to make vaccine seed material on 20 February. By early March, they had enough of it to start the manufacturing process. Clinical trials started 65 days after construction of the S DNA. The Oxford–AstraZeneca vaccine followed.[4]

More than 200 other vaccines against COVID-19 are under development using an extensive range of vaccine technologies, including traditional ones that use inactivated virus, and ones that use live enfeebled virus; the

Chinese inactivated virus vaccine CoronaVac has been widely used.

Vaccinators against COVID-19 have two aims: first, to stimulate immunity to protect the vaccinated individual, and second, to reduce the number of susceptibles in a population to such a degree that it massively reduces the ability of the virus to establish trains of transmission, maybe reducing the likelihood of their happening to zero, leading to its eradication. Current COVID-19 vaccines do the first very well. They have turned out to be more effective than even well-informed optimists dared to hope at the beginning of the pandemic; the Pfizer–BioNTech and Oxford–AstraZeneca vaccines give 92–98 per cent protection against mortality after two doses. The second aim goes under the rubric of 'herd immunity.'. This has always been a controversial term. When introduced in human medicine in 1929, it had a much broader meaning than it does today.[5] The British bacteriologists who first used it pointed out that 'there is little doubt that the English herd, as such, is immune to plague and to typhus' not because of the activity of its immune systems but because in England plague rats are very rare and lousiness is very uncommon.[6] Sheldon Dudley, who from 1941 to 1946 was Medical Director General of the Royal Navy, often used the herd word. His pioneering work on diphtheria in the 1920s and 1930s when he was Professor of Naval Hygiene at the Royal Naval Medical School at Greenwich showed the importance of immunization at the population level as well as the significance of new variants and of asymptomatic infections. He carried out this research on the 1,100 pupils at the Greenwich Royal Hospital School, a naval establishment. He was criticized in the House of

Commons for describing them in public as an 'experimental herd'. He defended himself vigorously, saying that biologically there is little fundamental difference between a herd of deer, a herd of swine or a herd of *Homo sapiens*. He called the antivaccinationists a subherd. In 1929 he said, 'They are ... perfectly honest in their convictions, but their power of dissociation and rationalization is so great that they often seem to the saner members of the herd to be absolutely unscrupulous and dishonest, whereas really they are only completely inaccessible to logic ... making the most absurd accusations against those who dare to differ from them.'[7]

At the time of writing, the pandemic continues, and it is far too early to predict how or when it will end. But the notion that global virus eradication could be achieved by herd immunity alone in its modern sense should be tempered by lessons from the history of other viruses, even after taking into account Adam Kucharski's aphorism, paraphrased, 'Once you've seen one pathogen ... you've seen one pathogen'. It had been calculated that the degree of herd immunity required for smallpox eradication was 70–80 per cent. Before 1967, the WHO eradication programme was based on this figure. In 1973 the 80 per cent goal had been achieved in India, but that year it had 88,114 cases. The WHO abandoned its herd immunity approach and moved to a programme of vaccination combined with case detection and containment, which controlled transmission even when vaccination levels were much lower than 80 per cent. It was successful. But inducing herd immunity sufficient to cause eradication did work for the lethal cattle disease rinderpest, caused by a virus related to measles. The key to success, extinction of the virus in nature, formally declared by the UN Food and Agriculture Organization in 2011, was a vaccine that protected against all virus variants, gave life-long immunity, was not associated with adverse reactions, gave immunity after a single dose, had a shelf-life of 30 days at room temperature, and had recipients who could not show vaccine hesitancy or become antivaxxers.

The thrombosis complication (vaccine-induced immune thrombotic thrombocytopaenia, VITT) associated with COVID-19 vaccines came as a big surprise. None of the vaccine components had properties previously known, or even anticipated hypothetically, to affect blood platelets or blood clotting. VITT is 10,000 times rarer than the thrombotic complications that occur in patients hospitalized with COVID-19.

A decline in protective immunity after vaccination and the need to revaccinate to restore maximum protection was not unexpected. Smallpox provides the lesson from history. Early vaccinators believed that vaccination immunity was life-long. But analysis of 680 cases arising from importations into Europe during the period 1950–71[8] found case fatality rates of 52 per cent in the unvaccinated, 1.4 per cent in those vaccinated 0–10 years before exposure to infection, and 11 per cent in those vaccinated 20 years or more before exposure.

12

Pandemics

COVID-19 is the first postgenomic pandemic. Only one other pandemic has begun in the Postgenomic Age, swine influenza in 2009. For all practical purposes, genomics passed it by; the UK stopped doing regular laboratory testing seven weeks after the arrival of the H1N1 virus from Mexico. But despite the importance of modern genomic sequencing, many aspects of COVID-19 natural history, public health control measures, and impact on society are not unique but hallowed by history. Quarantine dates back to 1403 in Venice.

The vigorous application of the postgenomic PCR tests means that we have a more accurate enumeration of the number of infections and mortality than in any previous pandemic. Even so, the frequency of asymptomatic cases means that guesswork has to be used to get the full picture.

But for the Black Death that struck England in 1348–9, it is all guesswork. Estimating mortality requires information about the population before the pandemic. But no population counts had been done between the

Domesday Book in 1086 and the introduction of the Poll Tax in 1377. So estimates of mortality have had to rely on indirect indicators, such as information about the number of deaths of beneficed clergy, and inquisitions *post mortem*, which were held to determine the heir to a land-holding tenancy vacated by death.[1] Neither gives information typical of the population as a whole, including of course, peasants, the majority.

In 2020, COVID-19 was very active in universities. The Black Death was also very active in universities, according to John Wyclif (Master of Balliol, 1361). He claimed that in the past there had been 60,000 scholars at Oxford, whereas now there were fewer than 3,000. The author of the standard history of mediaeval universities,[2] Hastings Rashdall, poured cold water on Wyclif's statement, holding that a much more credible estimate of student numbers before the Black Death was fewer than 3,000, a number claimed by city burgesses in their legal action after a Town and Gown riot in 1298, a count likely to be an overestimate. Rashdall excuses Wyclif by saying that 'the mediaeval mind was prone to exaggeration, especially where figures are concerned. It delighted in good round numbers, and was accustomed to make confident statements entirely without adequate data.' Rashdall was probably as right as anyone could be about student numbers, but was wrong about his temporal restriction of such a mindset. His characterization of the mediaeval mind fits Donald Trump's exactly, and applies regularly to other politicians in the COVID-19 era, and even, from time to time, to mathematical modellers.

Exaggeration and the very unsatisfactory nature of mediaeval records notwithstanding, there can be absolutely no doubt that the Black Death was very lethal, carrying off very important people; the Archbishop of Canterbury, Thomas Bradwardine, died of it on 26 August 1349, five weeks after his consecration.

It is far too early to speculate about any effects that the COVID-19 pandemic will have in years to come. But recovery from the Black Death seemed to be reasonably rapid. The long tradition at Oxford of bad relations between Town and Gown came to a violent head on 10 February 1355, a holiday celebrating the feast of St Scholastica the Virgin. A riot started in the Swyndlestock Tavern after a disagreement about wine between students and John de Croydon, the vintner. It lasted three days, causing the death of more than 60 students and much academic property damage. It is said that 2,000 peasants came into town from Cowley and other places to fight against the academics. A reasonable conclusion is that the peasant population had not suffered much more than decimation from the plague six years before. Elsewhere the mediaeval habit of founding new educational establishments continued, pandemic notwithstanding; the Universities of Perpignan and Huesca were established in 1350 and 1354 respectively, and at Cambridge, Trinity Hall was founded in 1350 and Corpus Christi College in 1352.

The cause of the Black Death, the bacterium *Yersinia pestis*, did not go away. Outbreaks came and went in England until the seventeenth century. In London the second biggest outbreak in that century occurred in 1625, with 35,417 deaths, and the last, and biggest, peaked in 1665 with 68,596 deaths. The disease then fizzled out. In 1666 only 1,968 died from it, and then there were fewer than ten cases annually until 1680, when no cases were recorded. Why it ended so suddenly is still an open question.

A third plague pandemic started in China in 1894, and was first recognized in Hong Kong in May. To investigate, the Japanese Government sent the bacteriologist Shibasaburo Kitasato and the pathologist Tanemichi Aoyama, and the French sent the bacteriologist Alexandre Yersin. Kitasato worked in a room in a plague hospital, and Yersin started his studies in a straw hut built for him in the grounds of the main hospital. Kitasato arrived on 12 June 1894, and by 14 June had found new bacilli in buboes (swollen inflamed lymph glands characteristic of plague – hence its appellation, bubonic plague), heart blood and internal organs from plague corpses. Yersin started work on 15 June and found new bacilli in the buboes of eight patients; he transmitted his findings to Paris where they were announced at a scientific meeting on 30 July. Kitasato and Yersin had discovered the plague bacillus almost simultaneously; it is named after Yersin because his description was more comprehensive and more useful bacteriologically. The timeline of their discoveries is uncannily similar to that of SARS-CoV-2 in Wuhan in December and January 2020. The next step in understanding the natural history of both pathogens was also similar. Food-borne transmission was top of the list of hypothetical routes for both; SARS-CoV-2 cases had a clear epidemiological link with the Wuhan wet food market. But the similarity soon disappeared. The COVID-19 food link was still-born. Not for plague. British, German, Austrian and Australian investigators favoured it. Traditional contagionist views also took hold, particularly after the spread of the pandemic to

India in 1896. Mortality peaked there between July 1904 and June 1905, with 1,328,249 deaths. It was thought that the bacillus became scattered around the surroundings of the sick and that it could enter the body through bare feet. Disinfectants were used on an enormous scale. Fresh air was considered to bring major benefits. It was observed that street beggars living in the open air seemed to be almost immune, whereas high-caste Brahmins living in houses with closed windows had high mortality rates. Comparison was made with the infrequency of infection suffered by prostitutes in London in 1665. As Procopius said in his description of the first pandemic in Byzantium in 542: 'plague is more deadly to saints than sinners'.

But modern accounts supplement Procopius by adding, 'only if the saints live in seclusion in rat-ridden homes'. The beggars avoided rat-infested houses, but the Brahmins had menageries of domestic animals.[3] Research in Bombay (now Mumbai) by the English Plague Commission started in 1905. More than 117,000 rats were dissected. The Commission found that bubonic plague was a disease of rats, that flea bites were necessary for it to spread from rat to rat, and from rats to humans, but in the absence of fleas, infection did not spread either from rat to rat or from human to human, even after the closest contact. Studies at the Lister Institute in London published in 1914 completed the epidemiological link. They showed that plague bacilli swallowed by a flea after biting an infected rat grow in the flea's proventriculus, the organ guarding the stomach, forming a mass big enough to block the further passage of blood. Hunger stimulates the flea to feed again. But the blockage stops blood getting into the stomach, and when the flea stops sucking there is a recoil. It causes the meal that the flea is trying to take to be regurgitated back into the wound, together with clumps of bacilli from the blockage. Fleas are very effective transmitters of infection because of this combination of injection and amplification. The key scientist in this study was Arthur Bacot. He excelled at growing fleas and lice, and spent more than a decade doing dangerous entomology, handling and dissecting infected insects. During the First World War he worked on trench fever, which he caught. He worked on typhus in Poland in 1920 and in Egypt in 1922, where he contracted the disease in his laboratory and died.

Knowledge of the routes of transmission of infection is an essential step in the development of effective control measures. Unfortunately, it is a topic much influenced by speculation and the application of 'common sense'. This is in part due to difficulties in conducting rigorous epidemiological investigations. Controlled trials present enormous administrative and ethical difficulties and are very rare. Volunteer studies on humans under carefully controlled circumstances have provided high-quality information in the past, but cannot be justified with pathogens that can cause untreatable lethal infections. Plague provides a good example, showing that the application of ineffective control measures, including ones that appear to be rational, can be harmful. In Bombay in 1897, measures focused on addressing environmental contamination and the finding of human cases and their isolation, because it was thought that plague was contagious like common infectious fevers. The Municipal Council employed 30,966 staff for the disinfection of houses and streets, and every day three million gallons of disinfectant were pumped into the sewers. But evidence emerged that flooding the drains with disinfectant drove infected rats into houses, with fatal consequences for their inhabitants. Popular resistance and rioting interfered with an isolation policy. Nevertheless, it soon became a well-known saying that a plague hospital was one of the safest places to be during the pandemic; doctors, nurses and visitors did not get infected by the plague patients. COVID-19 is very different. But there are similarities regarding disinfection policies, particularly the emphasis on hand sanitizing, which doesn't appear to be supported by any evidence that demonstrates its merit as an effective preventative measure.

As with COVID-19, the plague pandemic stimulated the development of state-of-the-art vaccines. Yersin had developed in principle a live avirulent one by 1895, and in 1897 Waldemar Haffkine started to manufacture one in Bombay using dead bacilli. It became a mainstay of plague control in India, and 40 million doses were administered during the next 40 years. It probably gave about 50 per cent protection. Antibiotic treatment made it redundant. Its place in history has been secured by the 1902 Mulkowal Incident. Plague had become common in the Punjab in that year and 505,849 people were vaccinated, 107 at the village of Mulkowal. Nineteen were injected with vaccine from bottle 53N. All developed fatal tetanus. The microbiologist Sir Graham Wilson, after reading the unpublished report of the commission that investigated the cause of the catastrophe, concluded[4] that the laboratory had been under heavy pressure to produce more vaccine, and that there had been a change in technique to make vaccine more quickly, a technical development with which laboratory staff were not familiar. Modern vaccine manufacture is far more complex and safer than in Haffkine's day. But the notion that it is just the speedy application of a formula derived from a patent, an impression that is left by the efforts of some campaigners who wish to increase SARS-CoV-2 vaccine production, is wrong. Lessons learned from Mulkowal, such as the absolute need for obsessional attention to detail regarding staff training, underpin the safety of modern vaccines.

Cholera has caused many pandemics. Currently we are in the seventh. Microbiologically it is easy to prevent. Human faeces must be prevented from getting into drinking water. The laboratory bacteriology of cholera has been straightforward since the discovery of its cause, *Vibrio cholerae*, by Robert Koch in 1883 (Nobel Prize, 1905). Glasgow escaped cholera in the fourth (1863–79) and fifth (1881–96) pandemics unintentionally because it had built aqueducts to supply it with water from a big clean highland loch, not to protect it from disease but for industry and fire-fighting.[5] Hamburg had no handy lochs of this kind and in 1892 had the last major cholera outbreak in Europe, ever.[6] Its unfiltered water supply from the polluted Elbe was notorious, as can be seen in this contemporary poem from a local newspaper (featured in Richard Evans's *Death in Hamburg*):

Of beasts in Hamburg's waterpipes
There can be found some sixteen types:
The lamprey, eel, and stickleback,
Of worms – three kinds – there is no lack.
Mussels three, slow snails the same

With jolly woodlice frisk and game,
A sponge, some algae, and a polyp,
through the sieve they jump and frolic.
As corpses in the pipes are found
The mouse, the cat, also the hound:
Unfortunately lacking yet –
The engineer and architect!

But Scotland didn't escape the third (1852–9). The appearance of cases caused alarm in Edinburgh.[7] Its Presbytery considered 'the propriety of appointing on ecclesiastical authority a day of prayers and humiliation' within its bounds, but went further. On 15 October 1853 its Moderator wrote to the Home Secretary, Lord Palmerston, asking that a National Fast be appointed on Royal Authority. Palmerston's lengthy but negative reply said that a law established by the Maker of the Universe 'connects health with the absence of those gaseous exhalations which proceed from over-crowded human beings, or from decomposing substances, whether animal or vegetable', and renders 'sickness the almost inevitable consequence of exposure to those noxious influences'. He concluded that:

> the best course which the people of this country can pursue to deserve that the further progress of the cholera should be stayed, will be to employ the interval that will elapse between the present time and the beginning of next spring in planning and executing measures by which those portions of their towns and cities which are inhabited by the poorest classes, and which, from the nature of things, must most need purification and improvement, may be freed from those causes and sources of contagion which, if allowed to remain, will infallibly breed pestilence and be

fruitful in death, in spite of all the prayers and fastings of a united but inactive nation.[8]

Palmerston's negative views on the epidemiological efficacy of prayer are at variance with the Moderator of the General Assembly of the Church of Scotland, Lord Wallace, who joined with other religious leaders in a call for prayer on 17 October 2021 in response to the pandemic.

Many millions died from cholera and plague in past pandemics, and the causative microbes have not gone away. But for more than a century it was the memory of influenza in 1918 that drove pre-COVID-19 public health planners. As the official UK Ministry of Health 'Report on the Pandemic of Influenza, 1918–19'[9] said, it was 'a pestilence which affected the well-being of millions of men and women and destroyed more human lives in a few months than did the European war in five years, carrying off upwards of 150,000 persons in England and Wales alone'. Superficially the number of deaths is similar to COVID-19 at the time of writing, and like COVID-19, the infections occurred in waves, the first in 1918 in June and July, the second from October to December, peaking in early November, and a third in February and March 1919. But most cases in the first wave were mild, unlike those in the second, which accounted for 75 per cent of deaths. The Report also said that 'the toll taken at the young adult ages of life is without any known West European or North American precedent', a fundamental difference from COVID-19. The Ministry of Health Report mortality table for London shows the ages of those killed by the virus: 46 per cent were aged between 25 and 45, and only 9 per cent were aged 65 and upwards. The report is illustrated with colour plates; Plate 2 'Illustrates a pronounced degree of the "heliotrope cyanosis". This patient is not in physical distress but the prognosis is almost hopeless.' And the Report says, 'in going round a large ward one could, without examining the patients at all beyond looking at their countenances, pick out those who were going to die with almost uniform certainty by reason of their colour alone'. In these patients the virus had caused pneumonia, and the lungs were filling with liquid. In 1918, fit young people were the hardest hit. US soldiers conscripted to fight in the First World War were better nourished and healthier than any other group of young men in the world, and they had all passed a medical examination. The history of the Medical Department of the US Army in the First World War[10] gives one of the most detailed records of influenza in 1918–19. Some 53.9 per cent of deaths from it were in soldiers aged 21–5, 1.23 per cent in soldiers aged 36–64. Across all ages it recorded 24,853 deaths from influenza, 469 from bronchitis, 10,341 from bronchopneumonia and 11,329 from lobar pneumonia – a total of 46,992. Most of the fatal cases of bronchitis and bronchopneumonia and many diagnosed as lobar pneumonia would have started as an influenza infection. The number of US Army battle deaths was 50,385.

The protective effect of masks was investigated. Some military camps in the US used them. Others did not. Of the 19 large camps that used them, ten had a below-average incidence of influenza, and nine an above-average incidence. Fifteen did not use masks, eight of which had incidences below average, and seven above average. It was concluded that general masking showed no benefit, a conclusion supported by results from Camp Custer in Michigan, where nurses were infected at a much higher rate than the average despite mask use being universal among them.

The First World War was drawing to a close when the lethal second wave struck. Histories of the war only mention influenza in passing. Its impact on the German army was proportionately much less than that of the US. The German Official Medical History of the war says that 1,531,048 soldiers died in battle, but that only 155,013 died of disease, including influenza.

On the US side, more than twice as many soldiers died from influenza in the US as in France. Being in the trenches in 1918 gave more protection from the pandemic than residence in a US Army Camp. Influenza in a US Army Camp again, but in 1976, had enormous ramifications for pandemic planners, because it led to the 'epidemic that never was'.[11] David Lewis was aged 18, and a recruit at Fort Dix, in New Jersey. He developed a respiratory infection on 4 February, but against medical advice went on a five-mile forced march. That night he collapsed and died. Influenza virus of the swine subtype was isolated. There were other flu cases in the camp. Four had the usual seasonal virus but three had the swine virus. Experts conferred. Their consensus was that the 1918–19 virus had come from swine, and that influenza pandemics happened about every 11 years. The last one was in 1968, so the time for another one was close. It was suggested that this new swine virus could kill one million Americans within the year. A press conference on 19 February run by CDC Atlanta, the national public health agency, mentioned 1918, and national TV that night showed archive stills from that year of people wearing masks. A 'Blue Ribbon Panel' of experts met with the President, Gerald Ford, in the Oval Office on 24 March. A vaccination programme for all Americans was authorized. It started on 1 October. Forty million doses were given, more than a million in the first 10 days of the programme. On 11 October three elderly people in Pittsburgh with a history of heart disease dropped dead at the same clinic shortly after being vaccinated. The local coroner appeared on national TV the next day. A body count started. President Ford and his family were vaccinated on TV on 14 October. The programme continued. At the end of November, six cases of the Guillain-Barré syndrome associated with vaccinations were reported; this is a paralytic complication that non-specifically follows a wide range of infections. The vaccination programme was suspended on 16 December. It never resumed. The virus never spread from Fort Dix. The Director of the CDC was sacked. The only epidemic was one of litigation initiated by people who claimed that they had suffered vaccination complications. And we now know that the 1918 virus came from birds, not swine, and that pandemics don't happen every 11 years.

When swine flu eventually arrived, in 2009, it did not behave as pandemic planners had predicted. Their considerations had been massively influenced by cases of bird flu, H5N1, in Hong Kong, which, although uncommon, were particularly lethal. The plans assumed that the next flu pandemic would be caused by a bird virus that would start in China or the Far East, that estimates of its lethality would be available before its arrival in the UK, that it would spread country-wide within one to two weeks, and that it would cause between 55,000 and 750,000 deaths. But the virus had not read the plan. It came from pigs in Mexico. It arrived in the UK four days after its initial identification. It spread unevenly in England and Scotland. It caused two waves; by the end of the second it had killed 457. Richard Neustadt and Harvey Fineberg were right when they entitled their 1978 'lessons-learned' report on the 1976 swine flu affair 'Decision-making on a slippery disease'.

Why influenza waves end so quickly has never been explained. Their termination has not followed the imposition of lockdowns or social distancing rules, because such things have never been tried during influenza pandemics, although to be fair to San Francisco, it had a law in October and November 1918 making mask-wearing compulsory in public places.

There is another UK COVID-19 parallel of a virus that hadn't read the plan, arrived from abroad, took off in the UK in spite of border controls, and had mathematical modellers taking centre stage in designing control measures which eventually needed the Army. Not only were the measures implemented without any cap on expenditure, they caused massive indirect negative effects on particular parts of the economy, costing the tourist industry at least £4.5 billion during the 9 months of the epidemic. The agent was the foot and mouth disease virus in 2001. The UK Contingency Plan was designed to deal with an outbreak of ten cases. By the time the virus was identified in February, it had spread to fifty-seven farms. Fundamentally different from COVID-19 in that it only infects ruminant animals, and that slaughtering the infected and contacts of the infected was the main UK control measure, nevertheless it could be said that slaughter is the epidemiological equivalent of human self-isolation and confinement in a quarantine hotel. Experience shows that the former is more virologically secure than the latter. If a rapid test had been available, far fewer slaughterings than 6,456,000 would have been needed. But at the beginning of the epidemic, the only UK laboratory allowed to handle the virus could only process 300 samples every year. Vaccines were available, but were not used, primarily for political and commercial reasons. A government policy of eradication at all costs, and the maintenance of all British herds in an immunologically virgin state, was set in stone, a policy going back to the Cattle Plague Act at the end of the 1860s. Walter Bagehot wrote about it[12] in words reminiscent of contemporary criticisms of current legislation about COVID-19: 'The details . . . may be good or bad, and its policy wise or foolish. But the manner in which it was hurried through the House savoured of despotism. The cotton trade or the wine trade could not, in their maximum of peril, have obtained such aid in such a manner.'

The Ministry with prime responsibility for controlling the 2001 foot and mouth disease outbreak was dissolved in March 2002. Public Health England had a similar COVID-19 role. Its demise and the reshuffling of its activities was formalized in April 2021. This was not a surprise. Repeated reorganization has been the fate of English public health microbiology. Public Health England was established in 2013. It replaced the Health Protection Agency, established in 2003, which in turn had replaced the Public Health Laboratory Service (PHLS), during the 'bonfire of the quangos'. The progenitor of the PHLS was set up in 1939 to deal with the epidemics predicted to follow Second World War bombing. Its most northerly laboratory was at Barnard Castle.

13
The Future

Are we going to have to live with COVID-19 for ever? Consider syphilis. It took off in Europe at about the time of Christopher Columbus's return from the New World. It remains the best guess that his sailors brought it back. A pandemic started. It continues. Sex is to blame. We have had to live with its causative spirochaete for more than 600 years.[1] An antibody test, the Wassermann complement fixation reaction (WR), was developed in 1906 and underwent massive scrutiny and refinement at international congresses run by the WHO precursor, the Health Committee of the League of Nations. Because it was not possible to grow the causative organism, *Treponema pallidum*, Wassermann and his colleagues used the liver of a foetus that had died from syphilis as the antigen source. It was soon found that extracts from normal liver worked just as well. In his detailed study of the sociology of the WR, Ludwik Fleck said that 'Wasserman and his co-workers shared a fate in common with Columbus. They were searching for their own "India" and were convinced that they were on the right course, but they unexpect-edly discovered a new "America".'² Fleck also pointed out that these discoveries started an avalanche of stud-ies; when he wrote about it in 1935, he estimated that WR work had generated 10,000 papers. The test has undergone many minor modifications, with a resultant effluxion of eponyms, but it is cheap, and not insensi-tive enough to be completely replaced by specific tests that use the organism (grown in rabbit testis), or by PCR looking for particular genes of the organism. A drawback is a specificity problem. Lepers are positive, as are some who have had a recent smallpox vaccina-tion. When applying years ago for a visa to work in the US, I took care to have my WR test before my smallpox booster jab. Official attempts to control the transmission of syphilis have all failed, exempli-fied by the massive 1887 oil painting 'Albertine in the Police Doctor's Waiting Room' by the Norwegian artist Christian Krohg, depicting prostitutes waiting to be examined for it, one of them, allegedly, painted by Edvard Munch. Luck struck, however, when Alexander Fleming (who, it is said, made lots of money treating sexually transmitted diseases, and didn't stay late at work but often visited the Chelsea Arts Club on the way home, possibly acting as a kind of medical adviser, which would explain why he had paintings by Wilson Steer and Philip Connard lining the walls of his Chelsea apartment) discovered penicillin, which kills the syphi-lis spirochaete as effectively today as it ever did, because its genome is so specialized and so trim that it lacks any sequences that could evolve into a resistance gene. The primary function of contact tracing is not to eliminate the spirochaete from the community but to identify people who need shots of penicillin into their buttocks. It is just as well that an effective treatment is available, because all attempts to make a vaccine have failed.

No drugs as effective as penicillin against syphilis have been found for COVID-19, yet. Interrupting its aerial transmission from person to person in the community can only be done effectively by imposing temporary lockdown measures that in themselves have detrimental effects. Wearing a face mask gives some personal protection against COVID-19, but probably less than wearing a condom does against syphilis, although judgement has to be reserved because the effectiveness of neither of them has been definitively evaluated in controlled trials. Will herd immunity eventually stop COVID-19 in its tracks? Will we develop an antiviral drug as effective as penicillin? Only time will tell.

Syphilis and COVID-19 are very different. Their differences illustrate the rule that every pathogen has its own individual strengths and weaknesses. COVID-19 is not influenza, but, unfortunately, pandemic plans in 2019 were directed against the latter. The concept of 'waves' of infection also comes entirely from influenza, even though mathematical modellers do not talk about them much because they have not been able to convincingly explain why influenza waves happen, why the Spanish flu had a low-mortality one in June and July 1918, a high-mortality one in October and November 1918, and a low-mortality one in February 1919. At the beginning of June 2020, I called myself a COVID-19 second-wave sceptic on this account, and because there had been no second-wave in China after its cessation of virus control measures, or one with SARS.[3] With the benefit of hindsight, I had been too optimistic about the effectiveness of contact tracing and case isolation, the response to and prevention of superspreader events, and the ability of border controls to prevent the importation of virus. In mitigation, in August I had drawn attention to the Leicester system of virus control used successfully against smallpox in the 1870s, which incentivized sufferers and their families to isolate by paying their wages, although it should be noted that the journal in which it appeared, the leftish *New Statesman*,[4] was not one likely to be heeded by the politicians presently in power in the UK.

Syphilis and COVID-19 have a major similarity, however, because for both, luck plays a big role in the outcome of an infection, an extremely common feature of many infections caused by bacteria and by viruses. In the pre-penicillin era, 30 per cent of syphilitics were unlucky, because years after their initial infection they developed serious complications. The spirochaete persists in all those who have been infected, but only in 30 per cent does it eventually take off in organs like the brain or major blood vessels to cause, in some, general paralysis starting with delusions of grandeur and ending with dementia, paralysis and death, and in others, an aortic aneurysm in which the main blood vessel behind the lungs swells up, burrows through the breast bone, and finally bursts. In the olden days, nurses at St Thomas's hung a big rubber sheet at the foot of such a patient's bed in preparation for this event. And for COVID-19, when the virus gets into a care home, about 30 per cent of the residents are lucky and only have an asymptomatic infection. The unlucky ones die. The outcome of infection in the residents, who nearly all have very similar risk factors, is fortuitous.

In the UK there is a long-standing tradition of responding to a catastrophe by setting up a Public Inquiry. Usually chaired by a judge, they are inquisitorial. Inquiry lawyers interrogate the participants, who also have their own lawyers, and the inquiry has the power to insist on the production of documentary and electronic evidence that it deems relevant. Hearings are held in public, with witnesses giving evidence under oath. The primary purpose is to establish the facts. It will also apportion blame; there has been debate about whether individuals receiving criticism should be warned before the publication of the Inquiry report to give them an opportunity to respond, a process that used to be called 'Maxwellization' because in the 1970s the late Robert Maxwell had vigorously complained about not seeing a draft report critical of his own activities. Calls for a Public Inquiry usually have a 'Lessons must be learned' theme.[5] Inquiries make recommendations. But the moment an Inquiry has delivered its report to the sponsoring Government minister, it ceases to exist; it has no standing. There is no legal obligation on the Government to implement its recommendations or if they don't, to explain why.[6] The 'Lessons to be learned inquiry' arising from the outbreak of foot and mouth disease in 2001 said that 'between 1922 and 1967 there were only two FMD-free years in the whole of Great Britain. Four epidemics were so severe that they prompted official Government reports in 1922, 1924, 1954 and 1968 ... There is a high degree of continuity in the central themes of these reports ... That is why we say that it is perhaps easier to identify lessons than to learn and act upon them.'

UK Public Inquiries take years and cost millions. I chaired one into a major *E. coli* O157 outbreak in South

Wales in September 2005.[7] We set out to be speedy and economical. Our inquiry took 3 years and cost more than £2 million. There was no Maxwellization. The main perpetrator had already been sent to prison. This inquiry was the second that I had chaired into an *E. coli* O157 outbreak; I concluded it by quoting Hegel: 'What experience and history teach is this – that people and governments never have learned anything from history or acted upon principles deduced from it.' The Prime Minister has said that a UK COVID-19 Public Inquiry will start in spring 2022, and Scotland's First Minister announced on 24 August 2021 that one north of the border would start earlier. Both will be chaired by judges, who were appointed in mid-December 2021. In the UK in recent times Public Inquiries have lasted on average about 30 months before reporting. It is reasonable to expect that the COVID-19 ones will be revelatory, even if many of the interested parties have for many months been anticipating them when writing minutes of meetings, preparing position papers, and being active in cyberspace. I hope that they will be asked about how they or their predecessors responded to the 2003 House of Lords Report[8] 'Fighting infection', which concluded that 'infectious disease services in England . . . are under-resourced and over-stretched . . . there is not enough surge capacity.'

It will also be interesting to read the comments of the inquiries on the mantra 'Following the science'. Don K. Price (adviser to President Kennedy) wrote in 1953:

Scientific methods are the most useful in determining *how* a specific thing is to be done: the more specific the thing, the more precise the determination. They are less often and less immediately useful in determining *whether* or *when* such things are to be done and *how much* effort or money is to be spent on them. But these are the controlling decisions, the decisions that must be made in the upper levels of the hierarchy if a government is to have any unity of purpose and action ... This relationship means, of course, that a much lower level of purely intellectual ability may be required for the decisions that come to the top of the government pyramid than for those that are made nearer the bottom.[9]

Failure to act on lessons learned does not apply to vaccines. Their manufacture, use and regulation have been massively influenced by the investigation of past adverse events and the application of methods to prevent their recurrence: in other words, sound science. In consequence they are very safe. The same principle has also been at work in intensive care units, where learning from the experience of treating COVID-19 patients has led to improved survival rates.

The US Supreme Court strongly disapproves of judges being involved in disaster inquiries because it thinks that they should not get involved in politics. Presidential Commissions do the job. If President Biden sets one up to investigate COVID-19 he will, correctly, be accused of engaging in pure politics.

The COVID-19 pandemic is the first postgenomic one. Whole genome sequencing and its offshoot, PCR, have been used on an unprecedented scale. That has not made it any easier to predict how the virus will evolve. It may get more virulent, or less virulent, or stay much the same. Mutants that enhance transmissibility have become common. Variants could appear that escape vaccine-induced immunity. The good news is that thanks to postgenomics, they will be identified quickly and new vaccines could be constructed with speed.

Along with the completion of unfinished business, in particular the worldwide eradication of polio, planning for the next pandemic has to be at the top of the agenda for virologists and epidemiologists. Predicting its cause or when or where it will start is impossible. The only certainty is that there will be surprises. Leprosy has been studied vigorously since its causal bacterium was discovered in 1873. But its recent discovery in African chimpanzees and British red squirrels was totally unexpected.[10] Is it yet another infection that came to humans from animals, like plague, and influenza, and arguably COVID-19? Bluetongue virus kills sheep. It is spread by midges. Its spread to northern Europe was predicted because climate change was leading to the northward spread of its main vector, the Afro-Asiatic midge, *Culicoides imicola*. Bluetongue arrived in northern Europe in 2006. But it wasn't a southern virus. It was a brand-new variant. And it didn't need *imicola*, because its vectors were local, indigenous midges.[11]

When the next pandemic happens, it will be detected and handled postgenomically. In the UK, COG-UK is setting up a national pathogen genomic service. In spite of the negative influence that the influenza model had on early attempts to control COVID-19, it must remain a prime pandemic possibility, with plenty of possible progenitors flying around the world in their avian hosts, promiscuously swapping bits of their perpetually mutating genomes more often than any coronavirus. Whether the appearance of a new virus with pandemic potential will lead to the peremptory imposition of lockdowns as an early preventative prescription, or whether pro-crastination is possible, will be a particularly pressing problem for public health practitioners, particularly in view of the unprecedented decline in respiratory virus infections, including influenza, linked to COVID-19-induced lockdowns.[12]

But park pessimism. Hans Zinsser wrote one of the plague literature classics, *Rats, Lice and History*, in 1934,[13] joining Boccaccio, Defoe and Camus but having the advantage over them of being a scientist who was a microbiologist and vaccine inventor. He said that it was a misconception that scientists are 'impelled to enter the career of investigating infectious diseases from a noble desire to serve mankind, to save life, or to relieve suffer-ing'. An example of this 'sentimental bosh' is that 'when a bacteriologist dies – as other people do – of incidental dissipation, accident, or old age, devotion and self-sacrifice are the themes of the eulogy'. Rather,

> it remains one of the few sporting propositions left for indi-viduals who feel the need of a certain amount of excitement. Infectious disease is one of the few genuine adventures left in the world. The dragons are all dead, and the lance grows rusty in the chimney corner. But however secure and well-regulated civilized life may become, bacteria, protozoa, viruses, infected fleas, lice, ticks, mosquitoes and bedbugs will always lurk in the shadows ready to pounce. About the only genuine sporting proposition that remains unimpaired . . . is the war against these ferocious little fellow creatures.

Notes

Foreword

1 R. Dulbecco, 'Basic mechanisms in the biology of animal viruses', *Cold Spring Harbor Symposia on Quantitative Biology*, XXVII (1962): 519–25.

2 Michael Billig, *Banal Nationalism* (London: Sage, 1995).

3 Nicholas Fraser et al., 'The evolving role of pre-prints in the dissemination of COVID-19 research and their impact on the science communication landscape', *PLoS Biology*, 19 (2021): e3000959.

4 T.H. Pennington and D.A. Ritchie, *Molecular Virology* (London: Chapman and Hall, 1975).

5 John Stuart Mill, *Nature, The Utility of Religion, and Theism*, 2nd edn (London: Longmans, Green, Reader, and Dyer, 1874).

1 The Postgenomic Age: Its Antecedents

1 Sarah S. Richardson, 'Race and IQ in the postgenomic age: the microcephaly case', *BioSocieties*, 6 (2011): 420–46.

2 Zunyou Wu and Jennifer M. McGoogan, 'Characteristics of and important lessons from the coronavirus disease 2019 (COVID-19) outbreak in China', *Journal of the American Medical Association*, 323 (2020): 1239–42.
3 S. Brenner and R.W. Horne, 'A negative staining method for high resolution electron microscopy of viruses', *Biochimica et Biophysica Acta*, 34 (1959): 103–10.
4 J.L. Heilbron and Daniel J. Kevles, 'Finding a policy for mapping and sequencing the human genome: lessons from the history of particle physics', *Minerva*, 26 (1988): 299–314.
5 Alvin M. Weinberg, 'Impact of large-scale science on the United States', *Science*, 134 (1961): 161–4.
6 Vaclav Smil, *Growth: From Microorganisms to Megacities* (Cambridge, MA: The MIT Press, 2019).
7 Paul Rabinow, *Making PCR: A Story of Biotechnology* (Chicago, IL: University of Chicago Press, 1997).
8 Angela N.H. Creager, *The Life of a Virus: Tobacco Mosaic Virus as an Experimental Model, 1930–1965* (Chicago, IL: University of Chicago Press, 2002).
9 Hugh Pennington, 'The problem with biodiversity', *London Review of Books*, 29 (2007): 31–2.
10 John White and Mark S. Bretscher, 'Sydney Brenner. 13 January 1927–5 April 2019', *Biographical Memoirs of Fellows of the Royal Society* (2020). Available at: https://doi.org/10.1098/rsbm.2020.0022
11 Lily E. Kay, *Who Wrote the Book of Life? A History of the Genetic Code* (Stanford, CA: Stanford University Press, 2000).
12 Horace Freeland Judson, *The Eighth Day of Creation: Makers of the Revolution in Biology* (London: Penguin Books, 1995).

13 T. Hugh Pennington, *When Food Kills* (Oxford: Oxford University Press, 2003).

2 Coronaviruses: The Beginning

1 David Tyrrell and Michael Fielder, *Cold Wars: The Fight Against the Common Cold* (Oxford: Oxford University Press, 2002).

2 Jenny Stanton, 'Blood brotherhood: techniques, expertise and sharing in hepatitis B research in the 1970s', in Ghislaine Lawrence (ed.), *Technologies of Modern Medicine* (London: Science Museum, 1994).

3 Dennis Rasschaert et al., 'Porcine respiratory coronavirus differs from transmissible gastroenteritis virus by a few genomic deletions', *Journal of General Virology*, 71 (1990): 2599–607.

4 Zunyou Wu and Jennifer M. McGoogan, 'Characteristics of and important lessons from the coronavirus disease 2019 (COVID-19) outbreak in China'. *Journal of the American Medical Association*, 323 (2020): 1239–42.

5 Cynthia S. Goldsmith et al., 'Ultrastructural characterization of SARS coronavirus', *Emerging Infectious Diseases*, 10 (2004): 320–6.

6 Roy M. Anderson et al., 'Epidemiology, transmission dynamics and control of SARS: the 2002–2003 epidemic', *Philosophical Transactions of the Royal Society of London B Biological Sciences*, 359 (2004): 1091–10.

7 Christophe Fraser et al., 'Factors that make an infectious disease outbreak controllable', *Proceedings of the National Academy of Sciences of the USA*, 101 (2004): 6146–51.

8 Myoung-don Oh et al., 'Middle East respiratory syn-

drome: what we learned from the 2015 outbreak in the Republic of Korea', *Korean Journal of Internal Medicine*, 33 (2018): 233–46.

9 Patrick C.Y. Woo et al., 'Discovery of seven novel mammalian and avian coronaviruses in the genus *Deltacoronavirus* supports bat coronaviruses as the gene source of *Alphacoronavirus* and *Betacoronavirus* and avian coronaviruses as the gene source of *Gammacoronavirus* and *Deltacoronavirus*', *Journal of Virology*, 86 (2012): 3995–4008.

3 COVID-19: The Disease

1 Hugh Pennington, Myrtle Street, *London Review of Books*, 23 (2001): 21–3.

2 Luke Milross et al., 'Post-mortem lung tissue: the fossil record of the pathophysiology and immunopathology of severe COVID-19', *Lancet Respiratory Medicine*, 10 (2022): 95–106.

3 Brian Hanley et al., 'Histopathological findings and viral tropism in UK patients with severe fatal COVID-19: a post-mortem study', *Lancet Microbe*, 1 (2020): E245–53.

4 Olivia V. Swann et al., 'Clinical characteristics of children and young people admitted to hospital with covid-19 in United Kingdom: prospective multicentre observational cohort study', *British Medical Journal*, 370 (2020): m3249.

5 M. van den Ende et al., *Chemotherapeutic and Other Studies of Typhus*, Medical Research Council Special Report Series No. 255 (London: HMSO, 1946).

6 Thirumalaisamy P. Velavan et al., 'Host genetic factors determining COVID-19 susceptibility and severity', *EBioMedicine*, 72 (2021): 103629.

7 RECOVERY Collaborative Group, 'Dexamethasone in hospitalized patients with COVID-19', *The New England Journal of Medicine*, 384 (2021): 693–704.

8 Matthew J. Burke and Carlos del Rio, 'Long COVID has exposed medicine's blind-spot', *Lancet Infectious Diseases*, 21 (2021): 1062–4.

4 Origins: December 2019–January 2020

1 Na Zhu et al., 'A novel coronavirus from patients with pneumonia in China, 2019', *The New England Journal of Medicine*, 382 (2020): 727–33.

2 World Health Organization, *Report of the WHO–China Joint Mission on Coronavirus Disease 2019 (COVID-19), 16–24 February 2020*. Available at: https://www.who.int/docs/default-source/corona viruse/who-china-joint-mission-on-covid-19-final-report.pdf

3 Hugh Pennington, *Have Bacteria Won?* (Cambridge: Polity, 2016).

4 Elizabeth W. Etheridge, *Sentinel for Health: A History of the Centers for Disease Control* (Los Angeles, CA: University of California Press, 1992).

5 Ibid.

6 Shannon E. Ronca et al., 'A 20-year historical review of West Nile virus since its initial emergence in North America: has West Nile virus become a neglected tropical disease?', *PLoS Neglected Tropical Diseases*, 15 (2021): e0009190.

7 Mary Douglas, *How Institutions Think* (Syracuse, NY: Syracuse University Press, 1986).

8 Lord Phillips of Worth Matravers et al., *The BSE Inquiry, Volume 1, Findings and Conclusions* (London: The Stationery Office, 2000).

9 Hugh Pennington, 'Host to host to host', *London Review of Books Blog*, 24 January 2020.

10 S. Burt Wolbach et al., *The Etiology and Pathology of Typhus: Being the Main Report of the Typhus Research Commission of the League of Red Cross Societies to Poland* (Cambridge, MA: Harvard University Press, 1922).

11 George K. Strode et al., *Yellow Fever* (New York: McGraw-Hill, 1951).

12 Mark Pallen, *The Last Days of Smallpox: Tragedy in Birmingham* (Mark Pallen, 2018).

13 T. Hugh Pennington, 'Biosecurity 101: Pirbright's lessons in laboratory security', *BioSocieties*, 2 (2007): 449–53.

14 Nicholas Wade, 'The origin of COVID: Did people or nature open Pandora's box at Wuhan?', *Bulletin of the Atomic Scientists*, 5 May 2021.

5 Fangcangs and Nightingales: February–April 2020

1 Simiao Chen et al., 'Fangcang shelter hospitals: a novel concept for responding to public health emergencies', *Lancet*, 395 (2020): 1305–14.

2 Hugh Pennington, 'Beware bad smells', *London Review of Books*, 30 (2008): 33–4.

3 Adrian Vaughan, *Isambard Kingdom Brunel: Engineering Knight-Errant* (London: John Murray, 1991).

4 Sarah Rafferty et al., 'Variola minor in England and Wales: the geographical course of a smallpox epidemic and the impediments to effective disease control, 1920–1935', *Journal of Historical Geography*, 59 (2018): 2–14.

5 Linda Bryder, *Below the Magic Mountain: A Social*

History of Tuberculosis in Twentieth-Century Britain (Oxford: Clarendon Press, 1988).

6 René and Jean Dubos, *The White Plague: Tuberculosis, Man and Society* (London: Victor Gollancz, 1953).

6 Test Test Test! March 2020

1 Ronald Hare, *The Birth of Penicillin* (London: George Allen and Unwin, 1970).

2 Hugh Pennington, 'Memories of the 1957 flu', *London Review of Books Blog*, 21 April 2020.

3 Hugh Pennington, *Have Bacteria Won?* (Cambridge: Polity, 2016).

4 Stephen F. Fitzgerald et al., 'COVID-19 mass testing: harnessing the power of wastewater epidemiology', *medRxiv* preprint. https://www.medrxiv.org/content/10.1101/2021.05.24.21257703v1

5 Stephen A. Brown, *Revolution at the Checkout Counter: The Explosion of the Bar Code* (Cambridge, MA: Harvard University Press, 1997).

6 Adam Kucharski, *The Rules of Contagion: Why Things Spread – and Why They Stop* (London: Profile Books, 2020).

7 Kenji Mizumoto et al., 'Estimating the asymptomatic proportion of coronavirus disease 2019 (COVID-19) cases on board the Diamond Princess cruise ship, Yokohama, Japan, 2020', *Eurosurveillance*, 25 (2020): 2000180.

8 Mohammad Rashidul Hashan et al., 'Epidemiology and clinical features of COVID-19 outbreaks in aged care facilities: a systematic review and meta-analysis', *EClinicalMedicine*, 33 (2021): 100771.

9 Daniel P. Oran and Eric J. Topol, 'Prevalence of asymptomatic SARS-CoV-2 infection: a narrative

review', *Annals of Internal Medicine*, 173 (2020): 362–7.

10 Myoung-don Oh et al., 'Middle East respiratory syndrome: what we learned from the 2015 outbreak in the Republic of Korea', *Korean Journal of Internal Medicine*, 33 (2018): 233–46.

7 The Epidemiologic Transition: Setting the Scene for COVID-19

1 Abdel R. Omran, 'The epidemiologic transition: a theory of the epidemiology of population change', *The Milbank Quarterly*, 49 (1971): 509–38.

2 S. Jay Olshansky and A. Brian Ault, 'The fourth stage of the epidemiologic transition: the age of delayed degenerative diseases', *The Milbank Quarterly*, 64 (1986): 355–91.

3 Kenneth Cowan et al., *Glasgow's X-Ray Campaign Against Tuberculosis, 11th March–12th April 1957* (Glasgow: Glasgow Corporation, 1958).

4 GBD 2016 Dementia Collaborators, 'Global, regional, and national burden of Alzheimer's disease and other dementias, 1990–2016: a systematic analysis for the Global Burden of Disease Study 2016', *Lancet Neurology*, 18 (2019): 88–106.

5 Vaclav Smil, *Growth from Microorganisms to Megacities* (Cambridge, MA: The MIT Press, 2019).

6 Min Gao et al., 'Associations between body-mass index and COVID-19 severity in 6.9 million people in England: a prospective, community-based, cohort study', *Lancet Diabetes and Endocrinology*, 9 (2021): 350–9.

7 Bruno Halpern et al., 'Obesity and COVID-19 in Latin America: a tragedy of two pandemics – official

document of the Latin American Federation of Obesity Societies', *Obesity Reviews*, 22 (2021): e13165.

8 Pinelopi K. Goldberg and Tristan Reed, 'The effects of the coronavirus pandemic in emerging market and developing economies: an optimistic preliminary account', Brookings Papers on Economic Activity Summer 2020, 161–211.

9 T. Hugh Pennington, *When Food Kills* (Oxford: Oxford University Press, 2003).

10 S. Jay Olshansky et al., 'Emerging infectious diseases: the Fifth stage of the epidemiologic transition?', *World Health Statistical Quarterly*, 51 (1998): 207–17.

8 Outbreaks: Learning in Real Time

1 Graham S. Wilson et al., *Topley and Wilson's Principles of Bacteriology, Virology and Immunity*, 6th edn (London: Edward Arnold, 1975).

2 Laura Ihm et al., 'Impacts of the Covid-19 pandemic on the health of university students', *The International Journal of Health Planning and Management*, 36 (2021): 618–27.

3 Jonathan W. Dyal et al., 'COVID-19 among workers in meat and poultry processing facilities – 19 states, April 2020', *Morbidity and Mortality Weekly Report*, 69 (2020): 557–61.

4 J.S. Haldane, *Report to the Secretary of State for the Home Department on an Outbreak of Ankylostomiasis in a Cornish Mine* (London: HMSO, 1902).

5 Lea Hamner et al., 'High SARS-CoV-2 attack rate following exposure at a choir practice – Skagit County, Washington, March 2020', *Morbidity and Mortality Weekly Report*, 69 (2020): 606–10.

6 Cho Ryok Kang et al., 'Coronavirus disease exposure and spread from nightclubs, South Korea', *Emerging Infectious Diseases*, 26 (2020): 2499–501.

7 Parag Mahale et al., 'Multiple COVID-19 outbreaks linked to a wedding reception in rural Maine – August 7–September 14, 2020', *Morbidity and Mortality Weekly Report*, 69 (2020): 1686–90.

8 Paul L. Delamater et al., 'Complexity of the basic reproduction number (R_0)', *Emerging Infectious Diseases*, 25 (2019): 1–4.

9 Kim Sneppen et al., 'Overdispersion in COVID-19 increases the effectiveness of limiting nonrepetitive contacts for transmission control', *Proceedings of the National Academy of Sciences of the USA*, 118 (2021): e2016623118.

10 Neal A. Palafox et al., 'Pacific voyages – ships – Pacific communities: a framework for COVID-19 prevention and control', *Hawai'i Journal of Health and Social Welfare*, 79 (2020): 120–3.

11 Mohammad Rashidul Hashan et al., 'Epidemiology and clinical features of COVID-19 outbreaks in aged care facilities: a systematic review and meta-analysis', *EClinicalMedicine*, 33 (2021): 100771.

12 Parham Azimi et al., 'Mechanistic transmission modelling of COVID-19 on the Diamond Princess cruise ship demonstrates the importance of aerosol transmission', *Proceedings of the National Academy of Sciences of the USA*, 118 (2021): e2015482118.

9 Whole Genome Sequencing

1 Simon R. Harris et al., 'Whole-genome sequencing for analysis of an outbreak of meticillin-resistant

Staphylococcus aureus: a descriptive study', *Lancet Infectious Diseases*, 13 (2013): 130–6.

2 Luke W. Meredith et al., 'Rapid implementation of SARS-CoV-2 sequencing to investigate cases of health-care associated COVID-19: a prospective genomic surveillance study', *Lancet Infectious Diseases*, 20 (2020): 1263–72.

3 Shuhui Song et al., 'The global landscape of SARS-CoV-2 genomes, variants, and haplotypes in 2019 CoVR', *Genomics, Proteomics and Bioinformatics*, 18 (2020): 749–59.

4 Louis du Plessis et al., 'Establishment and lineage dynamics of the SARS-CoV-2 epidemic in the UK', *Science*, 371 (2021): 708–12.

5 Ana da Silva Filipe et al., 'Genomic epidemiology reveals multiple introductions of SARS-CoV-2 from mainland Europe into Scotland', *Nature Microbiology*, 6 (2021): 112–22.

6 Joseph R. Fauver et al., 'Coast-to-coast spread of SARS-CoV-2 during the early epidemic in the United States', *Cell*, 181 (2020): 990–6.

7 Hugh Pennington, *Evidence to The Scottish Parliament Health and Sport Committee, ninth meeting of 2020, 28 April 2020.*

8 Dinesh Aggarwal et al., 'The role of viral genomics in understanding COVID-19 outbreaks in long-term care facilities', *Lancet Microbe*, 3 (2022): e151–8.

9 Dinesh Aggarwal et al., 'Genomic epidemiology of SARS-CoV-2 in a UK university identifies dynamics of transmission', *Nature Communications*, 13 (2022): 751.

10 Jemma L. Geoghegan et al., 'Genomic epidemiology reveals transmission patterns and dynamics of

SARS-CoV-2 in Aotearoa New Zealand', *Nature Communications*, 11 (2020): 6351.

11 Jemma L. Geoghegan et al., 'Use of genomics to track coronavirus disease outbreaks, New Zealand', *Emerging Infectious Diseases*, 27 (2021): 1317–21.

12 Courtney R. Lane et al., 'Genomics-informed responses in the elimination of COVID-19 in Victoria, Australia: an observational, genomic epidemiological study', *Lancet Public Health*, 6 (2021): E547–56.

10 Variants

1 William T. Harvey et al., 'SARS-CoV-2 variants, spike mutations and immune escape', *Nature Reviews Microbiology*, 19 (2021): 409–24.

2 Bin Zhou et al., 'SARS-CoV-2 spike D614G change enhances replication and transmission', *Nature*, 592 (2021): 122–7.

3 Emma B. Hodcroft et al., 'Emergence and spread of a SARS-CoV-2 variant through Europe in the summer of 2020', *medRxiv* preprint 2020, DOI: 10.1101/2020.10.25.20219063

4 Yang Liu et al., 'Delta spike P681R mutation enhances SARS-CoV-2 fitness over Alpha variant', *bioRxiv* preprint, 2021, DOI: 10.1101/2021.08.12.456173

5 Harald S. Vöhringer et al. 'Genomic reconstruction of the SARS-CoV-2 epidemic in England', *Nature*, 600 (2021): 506–11.

6 Baisheng Li et al., 'Viral infection and transmission in a large, well-traced outbreak caused by the SARS-CoV-2 Delta variant', *Nature Communications*, 13 (2022): 460.

7 Bo Meng et al., 'Altered TMPRSS2 usage by SARS-

CoV-2 Omicron impacts infectivity and fusogenicity', *Nature* 603 (2022): 706–14.

8 Lin T. Brandal et al., 'Outbreak caused by the SARS-CoV-2 Omicron variant in Norway, November to December 2021', *Eurosurveillance*, 26 (2021): pii=2101147.

9 Thomas P. Peacock et al., 'The SARS-CoV-2 variant, Omicron, shows rapid replication in human primary nasal epithelial cultures and efficiently uses the endosomal route of entry', *bioRxiv* preprint 2022, DOI: 10.1101/2021.12.31.4/4653.

10 Thomas Hugh Pennington, *Studies with Newcastle Disease Virus*, PhD thesis, University of London, 1967.

11 Robert Paul Hanson (ed.), *Newcastle Disease Virus: An Evolving Pathogen* (Madison, WI: University of Wisconsin Press, 1964).

11 Vaccines

1 K.A. Callow et al., 'The time course of the immune response to experimental coronavirus infection of man', *Epidemiology and Infection*, 105 (1990): 435–46.

2 Kizzmekia S. Corbett et al., 'SARS-CoV-2 mRNA vaccine design enabled by prototype pathogen preparedness', *Nature*, 586 (2020): 567–71.

3 Naif Khalaf Alharbi et al., 'ChAdOx1 and MVA based vaccine candidates against MERS-CoV elicit neutralising antibodies and cellular immune responses in mice', *Vaccine*, 35 (2017): 3780–8.

4 Sarah Gilbert and Catherine Green, *Vaxxers: The Inside Story of the Oxford AstraZeneca Vaccine and the Race Against the Virus* (London: Hodder & Stoughton, 2021).

5 Thomas Hugh Pennington, 'Herd immunity: could it bring the COVID-19 pandemic to an end?', *Future Microbiology*, 16 (2021): 371–3.

6 W.W.C. Topley and G.S. Wilson, *The Principles of Bacteriology and Immunity* (London: Edward Arnold, 1929).

7 Sheldon F. Dudley, 'Herds and individuals', *Journal of the Royal Army Medical Corps*, 53 (1929): 9–25.

8 Thomas M. Mack, 'Smallpox in Europe, 1950–1971', *Journal of Infectious Diseases*, 125 (1972): 161–9.

12 Pandemics

1 John Hatcher, *Plague, Population and the English Economy 1348–1530* (Basingstoke: Macmillan, 1977).

2 Hastings Rashdall, *The Universities of Europe in the Middle Ages, Vol. III. English Universities, Student Life* (revised and edited by F.M. Powicke and A.B. Emden) (Oxford: Oxford University Press, 1936).

3 L. Fabian Hirst, *The Conquest of Plague* (Oxford: Clarendon Press, 1953).

4 Sir Graham S. Wilson, *The Hazards of Immunisation* (London: The Athlone Press, 1967).

5 Hugh Pennington, *Have Bacteria Won?* (Cambridge: Polity Press, 2016).

6 Richard J. Evans, *Death in Hamburg: Society and Politics in the Cholera Years 1830–1910* (Harmondsworth: Penguin, 1990).

7 Thomas Ferguson, *The Dawn of Scottish Social Welfare* (London: Thomas Nelson, 1948).

8 Emendations from *The Life and Correspondence of Henry John Temple, Viscount Palmerston*, vol. 2, p. 265. London: R. Bentley, 1879.

9 'Report on the Pandemic of Influenza, 1918–19', Ministry of Health (London: His Majesty's Stationery Office, 1920).

10 Joseph F. Siler, *The Medical Department of the United States Army in the World War, Vol IX. Communicable and Other Diseases* (Washington, DC: US Government Printing Office, 1928).

11 Richard E. Neustadt and Harvey Fineberg, *The Epidemic That Never Was* (New York: Vintage Books, 1983).

12 Walter Bagehot, *The English Constitution* (Oxford: Oxford University Press, 1936).

13 The Future

1 Hugh Pennington, 'Can you close your eyes without falling over?', *London Review of Books*, 25 (2003): 30–1.

2 Ludwik Fleck, *Genesis and Development of a Scientific Fact* (edited by Thaddeus J. Trenn and Robert K. Merton) (Chicago, IL: University of Chicago Press, 1979).

3 Hugh Pennington, 'Fears about a second wave are unfounded', *Daily Telegraph*, 2 June 2020.

4 Hugh Pennington, 'Victorian quarantine, Letter of the Week', *New Statesman*, 14–20 August 2020.

5 Jo Goodman et al. (eds), 'UK COVID-19 public inquiry needed to learn lessons and save lives', *Lancet*, 397 (2020): 177–80.

6 Jason Beer et al., *Public Inquiries* (Oxford: Oxford University Press, 2011).

7 Hugh Pennington, *The Public Inquiry into the September 2005 Outbreak of E. coli O157 in South Wales: Summary*, 2009. Available at: https://

www.reading.ac.uk/foodlaw/pdf/uk-09005-ecoli-report-summary.pdf

8 House of Lords Select Committee on Science and Technology: Session 2002–03. Fourth Report. Fighting Infection. Available at: https://publications.parliament.uk/pa/ld200203/ldselect/ldsctech/ldsctech.htm

9 Don K. Price, *Government and Science* (New York: Oxford University Press, 1962).

10 Hugh Pennington, 'Red squirrels and leprosy', *London Review of Books Blog*, 13 December 2016.

11 Hugh Pennington, 'Short cuts', *London Review of Books*, 30 (2008): 21.

12 Djin-Ye Oh et al., 'Trends in respiratory virus circulation following COVID-19-targeted nonpharmaceutical interventions in Germany, January–September 2020: analysis of national surveillance data', *Lancet Regional Health – Europe*, 6 (2021): 100112.

13 Hans Zinsser, *Rats, Lice and History* (London: George Routledge, 1935).